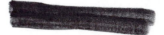

Muscular Analysis

of

Everyday Activities

Muscular Analysis *of* Everyday Activities

Elaine L. Bukowski, PT, MS, (D) ABDA
Associate Professor of Physical Therapy
The Richard Stockton College of New Jersey
Pomona, NJ

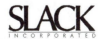

SLACK
INCORPORATED

an innovative information, education, and management company

6900 Grove Road • Thorofare, NJ 08086

Publisher: John H. Bond
Editorial Director: Amy E. Drummond
Editorial Assistant: April C. Johnson

Bukowski, Elaine L.
    Muscular analysis of everyday activities / Elaine L. Bukowski
        p. ; cm.
    Includes bibliographical references.
    ISBN 1-55642-462-0 (alk. paper)
        1. Physical therapy. 2. Motor ability--Testing. 3. Disability evaluation. I. Title.
    [DNLM: 1. Motor Activity--physiology. 2. Activities of Daily Living. 3. Muscle, Skeletal--physiology. 4. Physical Therapy--methods. WE 103 B932m 2000]
    RM701 .B85 2000
    612.7'4--dc21

                                                        00-041934

Printed in the United States of America.
Published by: SLACK Incorporated
                 6900 Grove Road
                 Thorofare, NJ 08086-9447 USA
                 Telephone: 856-848-1000
                 Fax: 856-853-5991
                 www.slackbooks.com

Last digit is print number: 10 9 8 7 6 5 4 3 2 1

DEDICATION

To my parents, Ed and Millie, for their encouragement to achieve any goals worth setting.

.....My heartfelt thanks!

CONTENTS

Section V: Upper and Lower Extremity Analysis

Section VI: Total Body Analysis

ACKNOWLEDGMENTS

Muscular Analysis of Everyday Activities is the result of 14 years of activity analyses presented and completed in the classroom. Numerous students have tested the techniques presented in the first chapter of this book and have been able to utilize and/or adapt them to their own analyses of daily activities. The data for the activities presented in this text have filled many notebooks and folders. This text has been in process for these past 14 years, both in mind and in heart. Thanks to the encouragement and support of my fellow faculty members and colleagues, Bess Kathrins, PT, MS; Thomas P. Nolan, Jr, PT, MS; Lee Ann Guenther, PT, MS; Mary Lou Galantino, PhD, PT; Winnie Welch, PT, MS; Patricia McGinnis, PT, MS; and Anthony Sgherza, PhD, PT, this text has become a reality. I also owe a debt of gratitude to all my current and former students who have either enthusiastically participated or have been dragged kicking and whining into the testing of this material. The challenges and stimulation they have provided me have been a driving force in getting this text written. The same can be said of all my former and current patients and clients; by not settling for second best, they pushed me to seek evidence to support the importance of their functional goals.

A special thanks to Michael Maggio, physical therapy student, who provided special assistance with the photography in this text. In addition, special recognition is due the Physical Therapy Department of the Bacharach Institute for Rehabilitation in Pomona, NJ. Their willingness to allow the use of their training car expedited the analysis of driving a car and the completion of the photographs for this analysis.

Through the support of all these people, my goal of transforming countless scraps of paper and stacks of measurements into a cohesive whole has become reality in the publication of this text.

ABOUT THE AUTHOR

Elaine Bukowski, PT, MS (D) ADBA, is a tenured associate professor of physical therapy at The Richard Stockton College of New Jersey, Pomona, New Jersey, and a practicing clinician at an outpatient physical therapy office. She holds a bachelor's degree in physical therapy from St. Louis University and a master's degree in anatomy, with a concentration in human gross anatomy and alternative educational teaching methods, from the University of Nebraska Medical Center. She is licensed by the state of New Jersey to practice physical therapy and is a certified senior disability analyst and diplomat with the American Board of Disability Analysts. The author's clinical experience covers more than 27 years in a variety of settings, including rehabilitation, oncology, home care, and outpatient physical therapy.

The author has worked in St. Louis Chronic Hospital and Cardinal Ritter Institute in St. Louis, Missouri; Holy Family Hospital in Berekum, Ghana, West Africa; Northeast Unit of the American Cancer Society in Philadelphia, Pennsylvania; Holy Redeemer Visiting Nurse and Home Health Agency in Philadelphia, Pennsylvania and Cape May County, New Jersey; Physical Therapy Services, Villas, New Jersey; Shore Memorial Hospital in Somers Point, New Jersey; and Maple Leaf Physical Therapy in Hammonton, New Jersey.

This is Elaine's fourteenth year of full-time teaching. She has taught courses in human gross anatomy, kinesiology, basic physical therapy examination and evaluation, and musculoskeletal physical therapy. She has also been an advisor and reader for student research projects, including such topics as resistive exercise techniques, sports prescreening, muscle strengthening techniques, normative values for range of motion in the elderly population, the use of acupressure and shiatsu in the treatment of low back pain, tai chi and balance, stretching techniques, exercise for patients with osteoarthritis, etiology of Achilles' tendinitis in runners, and the use of computer-based learning in human anatomy courses.

Elaine's own research projects have included studies on the use of guided experiences to increase student awareness of the importance of clinical skills, the teaching of ultraviolet, infrared, and diathermy in physical therapy curricula, the clinical measurement of spinal mobility in the well-elderly population, the reliability of measurement of range of motion by clinical observation, standard goniometer, and electric goniometer, the comparison of elastic resistance and free weights for increasing strength in wrist extensor muscles, and the comparison of the effectiveness of alternative educational methods in the study of human gross anatomy.

Elaine has published in professional journals and has chapters in *Disability Analysis in Practice: Framework for an Interdisciplinary Science* and *Physical Therapist's Clinical Companion*. She is also the co-author of a stereoscopic slide series for the self-study of human gross anatomy. She has presented papers and seminars, covering many different topics, at professional conferences on the local, regional, national, and international level, including the American Physical; Therapy Association, the Prosthetic and Orthotics Association of New Jersey, the American Physical Therapy Associations of New Jersey and Pennsylvania, the American Board of Disability Analysts, and the International Congress of the World Confederation of Physical Therapy.

Currently, she is involved in an assessment outcome study of an alternative teaching method for human gross anatomy in a physical therapy curriculum spanning an eight-year time period.

Elaine and her family reside in the southern part of New Jersey. She enjoys poetry, gardening, hiking, fishing, and music. She has published her poetry and is the composer of several pieces of music. She has a personal interest in complementary health care concepts and practices, in particular traditional Chinese medicine.

FOREWORD

Activities of daily living, or everyday activities, are the nuts and bolts that make up the tasks of an individual's day. Some of these activities, such as bathing, grooming, and dressing, prepare an individual for the day, while others are the tasks that are performed as part of one's day. Unless the ability to perform these activities of daily living is impaired, individuals pay little attention to the motions and the muscles that are responsible for the activities.

As academicians, rehabilitation professionals are faced with the task of educating students in the step-by-step analysis of activities that will enable the students to evaluate patients and clients and plan appropriate intervention programs based on their evaluation results. As clinicians, rehabilitation professionals are challenged daily to assist patients and clients in attaining functional outcomes through their rehabilitation programs.

Muscular Analysis of Everyday Activities was written as both a textbook and a reference source. This book was designed to facilitate observational, objective analysis of the performance of everyday activities. The materials presented in this book can be used by both students of physical therapy and occupational therapy, as well as by practicing clinicians in these two health fields. The analytical abilities fostered through the analyses contained in this book will provide a strong foundation on which students can build and learn to evaluate patients and clients. Practicing clinicians can utilize this material to confirm clinical findings, as well as plan intervention programs.

Selected everyday activities have been analyzed from the perspective of the types and amounts of motion needed to complete each task, as well as from the perspective of the muscles needed to produce the motions. Substitutions for the prime movers for all components of each task that was analyzed are included. In addition, suggested readings are provided to facilitate understanding of body motions and the muscles producing those motions, as well as multiple methods for analyzing body motions.

Section I

Introduction

Chapter 1

Performing the Activity Analysis

INTRODUCTION

Activities of daily living (ADL) include grooming, oral hygiene, bathing, toileting, sometimes with the use of personal care devices, dressing, feeding and eating, medication routine, health maintenance, socialization, functional communication, functional mobility, community mobility, emergency response, and sexual expression.[1] These activities enable individuals to get ready for their day and get themselves to their place of employment, school, and/or recreation.

The motions and muscular activity needed for all of the above are taken for granted until an injury or disease process occurs and interrupts one's ability to do the activity in the normal fashion. Each year at least 2 million individuals are hospitalized as a result of an injury. Injuries account for 10% of hospital discharges and 16% of hospital stays. Injuries sustained by those aged 15 to 44 result in 3.7 million years of lost life due to premature death and another 2.7 million years of lost productivity due to either temporary or permanent disability. For every person hospitalized because of an injury, nearly 25 people sustain injuries that, while not necessitating hospitalization, require medical attention.[2-3]

Physical therapists, physical therapist assistants, occupational therapists, and occupational therapist assistants, as students and practicing clinicians, are called upon to intervene and manage a patient's or client's case. This includes examining and evaluating a patient's or client's ability to perform a given activity. At first, this might seem overwhelming. However, if approached in a logical manner, the activity can be broken down into its component parts and readily analyzed.[4-6]

This chapter provides step-by-step procedures to analyze any given activity, both from a range of motion perspective and from a muscular perspective. As each step is presented, an example of a specific activity will be given so that the reader has a model to follow as he or she begins to analyze other activities of daily living.

One of the best ways to start any analysis is to observe the subject performing the given activity. View the subject from multiple angles (anteriorly, posteriorly, and laterally) and from multiple planes (coronal, sagittal, and transverse).[7-8] Be sure to view the subject from both sides, as one view could distort a movement better seen from another perspective. If possible, it is helpful to view the subject from above as well, as movements made in the horizontal plane can be missed from other views (Figures 1-1 through 1-5).

METHODS OF CAPTURING THE SUBJECT'S MOTIONS

Because a subject may tire while repeating the activity, consider one of the following imaging techniques to capture the motions of the subject.

A sequence camera is a method in which a series of eight photographs are taken at regular preset intervals. The interval set is dependent upon the velocity of the movement being analyzed. This is an inexpensive and easy to use system. However, the user is limited to eight photographs at set intervals.

Light pattern systems utilize lights attached at set anatomical landmarks. 35 mm cameras record a series of sinusoidal curves, while the subject moves along a marked trail. This is an inexpensive method of capturing a subject's movements. However, this system may be awkward to use, as the attached lights may interfere with movement.

Motion picture film is another method that utilizes the placement of markers on key landmarks. This method can provide frame by frame review, with fewer apparatus attached to the subject. It is more time consuming, more expensive, less available, and requires separate equipment to view and analyze the film.

Videography, or videotaping, also utilizes the placement of markers on key landmarks. Frame-by-frame review is possible, with fewer apparatus attached to the subject. It is less expensive, more available, and can provide immediate feedback to the videographer. This method can be time consuming but once mastered can provide quantitative data on a given subject.[9]

In addition, there are video camera systems that can be used with computer systems to capture, analyze, and print subject videos. Goniometric measurements, velocities, body symmetry, and sports activities can be obtained through the use of systems such as these.[10-16] However, these systems are more expensive than the conventional video camera.

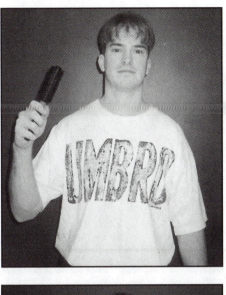

Figure 1-1. Anterior view of subject with a brush in the right hand.

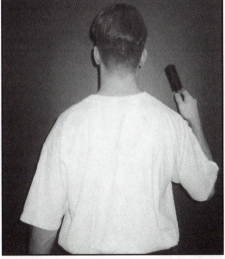

Figure 1-2. Posterior view of subject with a brush in the right hand.

Figure 1-3. Right lateral view of subject with a brush in the right hand.

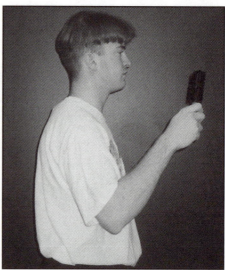

Figure 1-4. Left lateral view of subject with a brush in the right hand.

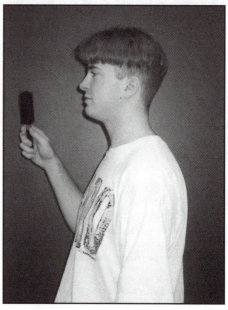

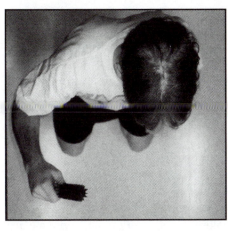

Figure 1-5. Overhead view of subject with a brush in the right hand.

Photography utilizing a 35 mm camera is another method of capturing a subject's motions. The photographer can capture given moments of an activity as the subject performs the activity. With this technique, the beginning and end motions within a sequence of motions needed to complete the activity must be established in order to ensure enough material to complete the analysis.

Videography offers several advantages over photography. The activity can be viewed in real time, whereas photographs provide a view of an activity at one given moment in time. Muscular activity is seen more easily on a videotape, because the subject is captured in real time, moving the body parts through motions. Goniometric measurements can be made from the videotape, provided a flat surface monitor is used to play back the videotape. (A flat surface monitor will not distort the angles of a given motion as the more common convex monitor will.) A video camera can be positioned unobtrusively, thereby not distracting the subject from his or her activity. Photographs require more posing to assure accuracy of angles and may therefore disturb the flow of the performance of an activity.

DETERMINING THE BEST LOCATION FOR BODY MARKERS

In order to calculate the range of motion of a particular body part, it is best to use some type of body marker.[17-23] Where to position the marker can be determined by viewing the preliminary videotape or photographs that have been made. Make a list of the motions that are occurring.

With this information, you can use the anatomical landmarks used for goniometry of these motions to set your body markers. These anatomical landmarks will allow you to calculate the range of motion occurring during a given part of an activity by providing specific points with which to align your goniometer.[24] For example, if you are viewing a subject who is brushing his or her hair, key body markers for the shoulder flexion motion would be the greater tuberosity of the humerus and the lateral epicondyle of the humerus. The marker on the greater tuberosity of the humerus would be used to align the axis of the goniometer, while the lateral epicondyle of the humerus would be used to align the moving arm of the goniometer. The stationary arm of the goniometer would be aligned with the subject's thoracic midline.

Once the best locations for your body markers have been decided, mark the subject. Self-adherent colored dots, masking tape with a black dot to indicate a point of reference, or washable body markers (Figure 1-6) can be used. For the spinal areas or rotational motions of the extremities, modified markers are helpful. An example of a modified marker is seen at the greater tuberosity of the humerus in Figure 1-6. This modified marker is made from a file folder label which has been bent in half and applied to the body.

Once the subject has been marked, re-videotaping or rephotographing of the subject can begin.

ESTABLISHING PHASES FOR THE ACTIVITY BEING ANALYZED

While doing the above, divide the activity into several phases which will facilitate the collection of all the data. For example, brushing the hair can be divided into the following phases: introduction and set-up, reaching for and grasping the brush, bringing the brush to the top of the head, stroking motions during brushing, and brushing the contralateral side of the head. This will enable you to establish a starting point from which the analysis is done and establish different starting and stopping points for capturing the subject's performance. This will also enable you to obtain goniometric data more easily and determine transitions in muscular activity more easily.

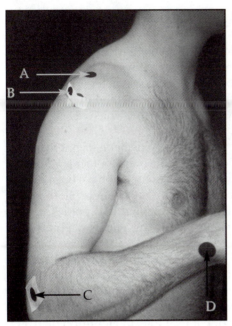

Figure 1-6. Examples of body markers: The marker on top of the shoulder (label A) is on the superior aspect of the acromion process; the marker immediately distal (label B) is on the greater tuberosity of the humerus. The marker on the lateral aspect of the elbow joint (label C) is on the lateral epicondyle of the humerus. The marker at the wrist joint (label D) is on the dorsal aspect of the head of the ulna.

VIDEOTAPING OR PHOTOGRAPHING THE SUBJECT WITH BODY MARKERS IN PLACE

Once the markers have been placed, have the subject perform the given activity while videotaping or photographing him or her again. Capture the subject's motions from an anterior and posterior aspect if the subject's motions include abduction and adduction. These are best visualized from this perspective. For motions of flexion and extension, right and left lateral views provide the best visualization of the subject's movements. Ideally, rotations are best seen from superior and inferior aspects. However, most facilities are not equipped to provide this viewing advantage. The next best views would be the anterior and posterior aspects for rotations. Have the subject repeat the activity at least three times while viewing him or her from these multiple angles. This will allow sufficient video footage or photographs from which the goniometric measurements can be taken.

DETERMINING GONIOMETRIC MEASUREMENTS

There are multiple ways of obtaining goniometric measurements of the body parts involved in a given activity. One way is to have the person freeze in a particular position, while the goniometer is aligned and a reading is obtained. However, this particular method involves many stops and starts, sometimes in awkward positions, which can contribute to errors in measurement.[25]

An easier way of measuring is using the videotape or photographs that have been made. With a videotape, pause the footage and obtain the goniometric reading using the body markers that have been placed on the subject. With photographs, be sure that enough photographs have been taken so that there is a beginning and end point for each motion being considered. Using the beginning and end points will enable a goniometric reading to be taken.

As mentioned previously, the anatomical landmarks that were selected prior to capturing the subject's performance on videotape or photographs become your key landmarks for taking goniometric readings. The goniometer can be aligned with these landmarks to calculate the range of motion that has occurred. For example, in Figure 1-6 there is a body marker on the greater tuberosity of the humerus and another body marker on the lateral epicondyle of the humerus. These two landmarks can be used to calculate the amount of motion for shoulder flexion.[24] To do this, the axis of the goniometer would be placed on the marker on the greater tuberosity, and the moving arm of the goniometer would be aligned with the midline of the arm, with its distal end aligned with the marker on the lateral epicondyle. The stationary arm of the goniometer would be aligned with the midline of the subject's lateral thorax. In this particular example, Figure 1-6 would represent the starting position for brushing the hair. A subsequent photograph would be needed to measure the ending position of the shoulder joint in that activity. By utilizing the starting position data and comparing it to the ending position data, the range of shoulder flexion can be calculated.

Another method for determining goniometric measurements is the use of a video camera system with hook-up to a computer system. Systems such as these calculate the goniometric measurements based on the data put into the computer system.[10-16]

VIEWING THE VIDEOTAPE WHILE THE ANALYZER PERFORMS THE ACTIVITY

Once all the goniometric measurements have been taken, the analysis of the muscular activity can begin. Play the videotape several times while performing the activity yourself. Feel what your muscles are doing as you move through each of the motions. Start with one particular joint and work your way up or down the body region that you are considering. Think about the forces that are at work on the body.[26-29] Is a concentric contraction or eccentric contraction needed? Does the body part have to overcome gravity or some external force, such as the weight of a tool or instrument, to move? If this is the case, the muscle will have to accelerate the body part to cause motion. However, if the body part needs to be controlled so that gravity or some external force does not overcome it, the muscle will have to decelerate the body part. In the former instance, the muscle will undergo a concentric contraction; in the latter instance, the muscle will undergo an eccentric contraction. If the muscle is performing a holding motion, an isometric contraction will be needed.

By now you realize this type of study of muscle activity will not be as easy using photographs, as the actual movements that are occurring cannot be seen. However, you can confirm your analysis by palpating the subject's muscles as the subject performs the activity. (Obviously, the deeper lying muscles will be harder to palpate.) You can still perform the activity yourself and do the same type of muscular analysis as listed above. In this way, you can make comparisons between what you palpated and what you obtained by performing the activity yourself.

Another method of muscle analysis is the use of electromyography. This can be accomplished with the use of surface electrodes or fine portable or lab type wire. Care must be taken to insure that the recording mechanisms, either surface electrodes or fine wire, are placed at key motor points to secure data. As with any instrument used to record data, there are disadvantages that need to be considered. For instance, when using surface electrodes, the area from which the recording is made is relatively large and the recording will represent only superficial muscles. When using implanted fine wire electrodes, there may be subject discomfort with puncture of the skin during insertion, a tendency for the wires to migrate within the muscle, and possible microtrauma to the tissues if this movement is not minimized. For further information on the use of electromyography, the reader is referred to Soderberg and Cook's article in the December 1984 issue of *Physical Therapy*; Soderberg's text on kinesiology; Robinson and Snyder-Mackler's text on clinical electrophysiology; and Nelson and Currier's text on clinical electrotherapy.[30-33]

DETERMINING THE MUSCULAR ACTIVITY OF THE SUBJECT

Once this initial muscular analysis has been completed, you are now ready to view the videotape or the photographs again and start listing the muscular activity needed to perform the motions being done by the subject. Particular attention should be focused on the forces acting upon the subject throughout the activity. This will help determine and/or confirm the specific type of muscular contraction needed.[26-29] If electromyography was used during the time you captured your subject's performance on videotape or photographic film, the muscular analysis is determined from the data collected by the system used.

Having performed the activity yourself, you can begin to compare the subject's performance to your own. This will alert you to the possibility of muscle substitution, either by your subject or yourself. If muscles are being substituted for any movements, you will have a starting point for the intervention you need to employ for your subject.

PUTTING IT ALL TOGETHER

By the end of all these steps, you will have accumulated a substantial amount of data about the subject. This data can be organized in chart form for a visual presentation or for a written presentation. Tables 1-1 and 1-2 contain examples of chart presentations of selected goniometric measurements and primary muscle activity for joint motions involved in brushing the hair.

A summary of the steps taken to get to the written presentation follows:

1) Have subject perform the activity while you observe.

2) Make a list of the motions that are occurring.

3) Determine the anatomical landmarks used for goniometry of these motions.

4) Determine the location of your body markers based on these anatomical landmarks.

5) Divide the activity into phases.

Table 1-1
Goniometric Measurements for Reaching for the Brush

Joint	Motion	Degrees of Movement
Shoulder	Flexion	0 to 50
Elbow	Extension	No motion occurring
Radioulnar	Pronation	0 to 23
Wrist	Extension	0 to 15
Ulnar	Deviation	0 to 10

Example of a chart presentation of goniometric measurements.

Table 1-2
Upper Extremity Primary Muscles Used in Brushing the Hair

Joint	Motion	Normal Muscles
Shoulder	Flexion	Anterior deltoid, coraco-brachialis, pectoralis major
	Extension	Same as above
	Horizontal abduction	Posterior deltoid
	Horizontal adduction	Pectoralis major
	External rotation	Infraspinatus, teres minor
	Internal rotation	Subscapularis, pectoralis major, latissimus dorsi, teres major
Elbow	Flexion	Biceps brachii, triceps brachii (acting eccentrically)
	Extension	Triceps brachii
Forearm	Pronation	Pronator teres, pronator quadratus
	Supination	Biceps brachii, supinator

continued on next page

Table 1-2 (continued)
Upper Extremity Primary Muscles Used in Brushing the Hair

Joint	Motion	Normal Muscles
Wrist	Extension	Extensors carpi radialii longus, brevis, and ulnaris
	Ulnar deviation	Extensor carpi ulnaris, flexor carpi ulnaris
	Radial deviation	Flexor carpi radialis, extensors carpi radialii longus and brevis

Example of a chart presentation of primary muscle activity.

6) Position the body markers on your subject.

7) Have subject perform the activity again while you capture the performance with the method you have chosen (video tape, photographs, etc).

8) Calculate the goniometric measurements for the motions of the activity.

9) Calculate the muscular activity.

By following the above procedures, you will have a logical way of performing a muscular analysis for any given activity. In the following chapters, examples of specific muscular analyses are presented. These analyses include the range of motion needed to complete an activity, as well as the muscles utilized in performing the activity.

Photography was the method used to capture the subject's performance of each activity. Observational analysis, along with palpatory techniques, was the method used to determine the muscular activity. These methods were chosen because they are commonly employed in clinical settings.

Each subsequent chapter concludes with a summary of the key anatomical landmarks used for the analysis, a summary of the major phases for the analysis, a summary of the joint motions and muscular activity, and a clinical application and discussion question section to foster further analyses. Suggested readings are provided to lead the reader to other materials that deal with information on muscular analyses.

Section II focuses on the use of the upper extremity in selected activities of daily living. In most of these activities, the more proximal components of an extremity serve the more distal components by positioning and stabilizing the extremity in space. Therefore, it may appear that greater attention has been directed to the more distal components, when in reality, all components of the extremity were analyzed based on the work being done by each. Although the lower extremity and the spine are involved in activities, the upper extremity was chosen as the focal point for the first several analyses. Subsequent sections of the book focus on the use of the lower extremity and the use of the back, thereby helping the reader to focus on these areas of the body one by one. Section V is devoted to combining an analysis of both the upper and lower extremities to assist the reader in building toward a total body analysis, which is presented in section VI.

Such an approach was used to avoid overwhelming the reader with the vast amounts of data that can be collected during a total body analysis. By doing so, the reader can build confidence in choosing appropriate landmarks for body markers and appropriate viewing angles to complete a goniometric and muscular analysis of the activities presented. The reader can work toward total body analysis as he or she applies anatomical and kinesiological knowledge to increasing amounts of joint motions and muscular activities.

CLINICAL APPLICATION AND DISCUSSION QUESTIONS

This chapter presented an overview of different methods for analyzing any activity. Whether observation, photography, videography, and/or computerized systems are used to analyze a subject's activity, establishing key anatomical landmarks at the onset is a common thread to any muscular analysis.

Do an analysis of the upper extremity while a subject is reaching for a book on an overhead shelf. To help you get started, follow these steps:

1) Define the starting position for this activity.

2) Do the activity yourself and decide how you will break the activity into significant phases for analysis.

3) Determine the appropriate anatomical landmarks that you will use to calculate the range of motion of the upper extremity joints.

4) Determine the appropriate angles from which to view a subject to analyze the above activity.

5) Choose a subject and place appropriate stickers on the anatomical landmarks that are key to this analysis.

6) Choose a method for recording the analysis. For example, photograph your subject.

7) Use the anatomical landmarks on the photographs and calculate the range of motion at each of the key joints. Record this data.

8) Determine the muscles that are the prime movers at each key joint.
   a) Do the activity yourself and feel what muscles are active at the key joints.
   b) Have your subject do the activity again and observe the muscular activity. You may have to palpate the subject to feel the muscles.
   c) Record the muscular activity at the key joints.

9) Collate the data you collected. You can use charts or tables to assemble your data. See Tables 1-1 and 1-2 for examples of charting your data.

REFERENCES

1. Lamport NK, Coffey MS, Hersch GI. *Activity Analysis and Application: Building Blocks of Treatment*. 3rd ed. Thorofare, NJ: SLACK Inc; 1996.
2. Max W, Rice DP, MacKenzie EJ. The lifetime cost of injury. *Inquiry*. 1990;27:332-343.
3. Brody JE. For artists and musicians creativity can mean illness and injury. *New York Times*, October 17, 1989.
4. Viano DC, King AI, Melvin JW, Weber K. Injury biomechanics research: an essential element in the prevention of trauma. *J Biomech*. 1989;22:403-417.
5. Huss J. From kinesiology to adaptation. *Am J Occup Ther*. 1981;35:574-580.
6. Licht S. Kinetic analysis of crafts and occupations. *Occup Ther and Rehabil*. 1947;26:75-78.
7. Drury C. Task analysis methods in industry. *Appl Ergonomics*. 1983;14:19-28.

8. Wei SH, McQuade KJ, Smidt GL. Three-dimensional joint range of motion measurements from skeletal coordinate data. *J Ortho Sports Phys Ther.* 1993;18:687-691.

9. Pedersen E, Klemar B. Recording of physiological measurements based on video technique. *Scand J Rehabil Med.* 1974;3(suppl):45-50.

10. Bruegger W, Milner M. Computer-aided tracking of body motions using a CCD image sensor. *Med Biol Eng Comput.* 1978,16.207-210.

11. Klein PJ, Dehaven JJ. Accuracy of three dimensional linear and angular estimates obtained with Ariel Performance Analysis System.™ *Arch Phys Med Rehabil.* 1995;76:183-189.

12. Scholz JP. Reliability and validity of the WATSMART™ three-dimensional optoelectric motion analysis system. *Phys Ther.* 1989;69:679-689.

13. Scholz JP, Millford JP. Accuracy and precision of the Peak™ performance technologies motion measurement system. *J Motor Behav.* 1993;25:2-7.

14. VanderLinden DW, Carlson SJ, Hubbard RL. Reproducibility and accuracy of angle measurements obtained under static conditions with the Motion Analysis™ video system. *Phys Ther.* 1992;72:300-305.

15. Wilson DJ, Smith BK, Gibson JK. Accuracy of reconstructed angular estimates obtained with the Ariel Performance Analysis System.™ *Phys Ther.* 1997;77:1741-1746.

16. Hubbard M. Computer simulation in sport and industry. *J Biomech.* 1993;26(suppl 1):53-61.

17. An KN, Chao EYS. Kinematic analysis of human movement. *Ann Biomed Eng.* 1984;12:585-597.

18. Kinzel GL, Hall AS, Hillberty BM. Measurement of the total motion between two body segments - 1. Analytical development. *J Biomech.* 1972;5:93-105.

19. Simon SR, Nuzzo RM, Koskinen MM. A comprehensive clinical system for four dimensional motion analysis. *Bull Hosp Jt Dis.* 1977;38:41-44.

20. Spoor CW, Veldpaus FE. Rigid body motion calculated from spatial coordinates of markers. *J Biomech.* 1980;13:391-393.

21. Söderkvist I, Wedin PA. Determining the movements of the skeleton using well-conditioned markers. *J Biomech.* 1993;58:426-432.

22. Soechting JF, Flanders M. Moving in three-dimensional space: frames of reference, vectors, and coordinate systems. *Annu Rev Neurosci.* 1992;15:167-191.

23. Sommer JH, Miller NR. A technique for kinematic modeling of anatomical joints. *J Biomech Eng.* 1980;102:311-317.

24. Norkin CC, White DJ. *Measurement of Joint Motion—A Guide to Goniometry.* 2nd ed. Philadelphia, Pa: FA Davis Co; 1995.

25. Boone DC, Azen SP, Lin CM, Spence C, Bacon C, Lee L. Reliability of goniometric measurements. *Phys Ther.* 1978;58:1355-1390.

26. Bigland B, Lippold OCJ. The relation between force, velocity, and integrated electrical activity in human muscles. *J Physiol.* 1954;123:214-224.

27. Zajac FE, Gordon ME. Determining muscle force and action in multiarticular movement. *Exerc Sport Sci Rev.* 1989;17:187-230.
28. Knapik JJ, Wright JE, Mawdsley RH, Braum J. Isometric, isotonic, and isokinetic torque variations in four muscle groups through a range of joint motion. *Phys Ther.* 1983;63:938-947.
29. Stauber WT. Eccentric action muscles: physiology, injury, and adaptation. *Exerc Sport Sci Rev.* 1989;17:157-185.
30. Soderberg GL, Cook TM. Electromyography in biomechanics. *Phys Ther.* 1984;12:1813-1820.
31. Soderberg GL. *Kinesiology—Application to Pathological Motion.* Baltimore, Md: Williams & Wilkins; 1986.
32. Robinson AJ, Snyder-Mackler L. *Clinical Electrophysiology—Electrotherapy and Electrophysiological Testing.* 2nd ed. Baltimore, Md: Williams & Wilkins; 1995.
33. Nelson RM, Currier DP. *Clinical Electrotherapy.* 2nd ed. Norwalk, Conn: Appleton & Lange; 1991.

SUGGESTED READINGS

Adams MAP, Dolan CM, Hutton WC. An electronic inclinometer technique for measuring lumbar curvature. *Clin Biomech.* 1986;1:130-134.

Altman DG, Bland JM. Measurement in medicine: the analysis of method comparison studies. *Statistician.* 1983;32:307-317.

Aptekar RG, Ford F, Bleck EE. Light patterns as a means of assessing and recording gait. I. Methods and results in normal children. *Dev Med Child Neurol.* 1976;18:31-36.

Ayoub MM. Human movement recording for biomechanical analysis. *International Journal of Product Research.* 1972;10:35-51.

Baolgun JA, Abereoje OK, Olaogun MO, Obajuluwa VA. Inter- and intratester reliability of measuring neck motions with tape measure and Myrin gravity reference goniometer. *J Orthop Sports Phys Ther.* 1989;10:248-253.

Chaffin DB. A computerized biomechanical model development of and use in studying gross body actions. *J Biomech.* 1969;2:429-441.

Chao EYE. Justification of triaxial goniometer for the measurement of joint rotation. *J Biomech.* 1980;13:989-1006.

Edelman S, Flash T. A model of handwriting. *Biol Cybern.* 1987;57:25-36.

Foley CD, Quanbury AO, Steinke T. Kinematics of normal child locomotion—a statistical study based on TV data. *J Biomech.* 1979;12:1-16.

Gauvin MC, Riddle DL, Rothstein JM. Reliability of clinical measurements of forward bending using the modified fingertip-to-floor method. *Phys Ther.* 1990;70:443-447.

Haggard P, Wing AM. Assessing and reporting the accuracy of position measurement made with optical tracking systems. *J Motor Behav.* 1990;22:315-321.

Holt KS, Jones RB, Wilson R. Gait analysis by means of a multiple sequential exposure camera. *Dev Med Child Neurol.* 1974;16:742-745.

Madson TJ, Youdas JW, Suman VJ. Reproducibility of lumbar spine range of motion measurements using the back range of motion device. *J Orthop Sports Phys Ther.* 1999;29:470-477.

Mayer TG, Kondraske G, Beals SB, Gatchel RJ. Spinal range of motion. Accuracy and sources of error with inclinometric measurement. *Spine.* 1997;22:1976-1984.

Merritt JL, McLean TJ, Erichson RP, Offord KP. Measurement of trunk flexibility in normal subjects: reproducibility of three clinical methods. *Mayo Clin Proc.* 1986;61:192-197.

Morris JRW. Accelerometry—a technique for the measurement of human body movements. *J Biomech.* 1973;6:729-736.

Nawoczenski DA, Baumhauer JF, Umberger BR. Relationship between clinical measurements and motion of the first metatarsophalangeal joint during gait. *J Bone Joint Surg Am.* 1999;81:370-376.

Pearcy MJ, Gill JM, Whittle MW, Johnson GR. Dynamic back movement measured using a three-dimensional television system. *J Biomech.* 1987;20:943-949.

Pearcy MJ, Hindle RJ. New method for the non-invasive three-dimensional measurement of human back movement. *Clin Biomech.* 1989;4:73-79.

Pearcy M, Portek I, Shepherd J. Three-dimensional X-ray analysis of normal movement in the lumbar spine. *Spine.* 1984;9:294-297.

Persson T, Lanshammar H, Medved V. A marker-free method to estimate joint center of rotation by video image processing. *Comput Meth Programs Biomed.* 1995;46:217-224.

Rheault W, Ferris S, Foley JA, Schaffauser D, Smith R. Intertester reliability of the flexible ruler for the cervical spine. *J Orthop Sports Phys Ther.* 1989;10:254-256.

Smidt GL, Day JW, Gerleman DG. Iowa anatomical position system. A method of assessing posture. *Eur J Appl Physiol.* 1984;52:407-413.

Taylor CL, Blaschke AC. A method of kinematic analysis of the shoulder, arm, and hand complex. *Ann N Y Acad Sci.* 1951;51:1251-1265.

Van Zuylen EJ, Gielen AM, Van Der Gon JJD. Coordination and inhomogenous activation of human arm muscles during isometric torques. *J Neurophys.* 1988;60:1523-1548.

Woltring HJ. Representation and calculation of 3-D joint movement. *Human Movement Science.* 1991;10:603-616.

Woltring HJ. 3-D attitude representation of human joints: a standardization proposal. *J Biomech.* 1994;27:1399-1414.

Youdas JW, Carey JR, Garrett TR. Reliability of measurements of cervical spine range of motion—comparison of three methods. *Phys Ther*. 1991;71:98-104.

Youdas JW, Suman VJ, Garrett TR. Reliability of measurements of lumbar spine sagittal mobility obtained with the flexible curve. *J Orthop Sports Phys Ther*. 1995;21:13-20.

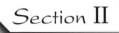

Section II

Upper Extremity
Analyses

Chapter 2

Shaving the Face

INTRODUCTION AND SET-UP

The upper extremity is extremely important to the activity of shaving the face with a conventional (nonelectric) razor. This activity was analyzed from the following perspective: the shaving cream had been placed on the face, and the razor blade was in its holder. The subject was standing in the anatomical position in front of a washstand, with a mirror above it, on which the razor was positioned. The 5-inch razor was situated 4 inches from the edge of the 30-inch high washstand (Figure 2-1). In order to shave the face, the individual had to complete the following three steps in sequence: first, the individual had to reach for and grasp the razor; next, the individual needed to bring the razor to the face; and finally, the individual performed the stroking motions needed to complete the actual shaving aspect of this activity.

Based on the above sequencing of events, it became apparent that most, if not all, of the joints of the upper extremity were involved in this activity. One of the most important areas of the body involved in shaving the face was the shoulder complex, which helped position the rest of the upper extremity in space for function to occur.[1] This complex consists of the sternoclavicular, acromioclavicular, scapulothoracic, and glenohumeral joints.[2-9] It comprises approximately 25% to 50% of the weight of the entire upper extremity. The elbow complex, consisting of the humeroulnar, humeroradial, and superior and inferior radioulnar joints, serves a similar function to help position the more distal wrist and hand in space.[10-13] The wrist complex, formed by the radiocarpal and midcarpal joints, further serves the hand by positioning it in space and creating a good length-tension relationship for the muscles that control the movements of the hand.[14-22] Finally, the carpometacarpal (CMC), metacarpophalangeal (MCP), and interphalangeal (IP) joints of the hand manipulated the razor, enabling the activity to be completed.[23-27]

Figure 2-1. Starting position: Subject and razor in place. The key landmarks denoted by black dots are: A = acromion process (dorsal aspect); B = greater tuberosity of humerus; C = lateral epicondyle of humerus; D = ulnar head (dorsal aspect); E = radial styloid process (dorsal aspect); F = radial styloid process (radial aspect); and G = first MCP joint line (radial aspect).

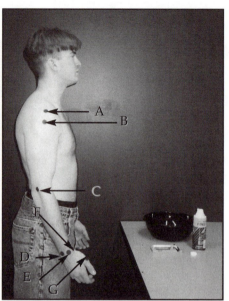

To facilitate the analysis of this activity of daily living, each joint of the upper extremity was analyzed individually.

The shoulder complex, which was working throughout the entire task of shaving, provided the smoothest and greatest range of motion possible to the upper extremity. The glenohumeral joint alone would have been unable to perform a full range of shoulder abduction or flexion. The remainder of the range was provided by the scapulothoracic, sternoclavicular, and acromioclavicular joints. The specific contributions made by these joints is referred to as scapulohumeral rhythm.[4,28-31]

Scapulohumeral rhythm is the overall ratio of 2 degrees of glenohumeral motion to one degree of scapulothoracic motion to reach a maximum range of elevation of 180 degrees. The achievement of this maximum range is important. More relevant to the activity of shaving is the ability of this rhythm to maintain the glenoid fossa in an optimal position to receive the head of the humerus and maintain a good length-tension relationship for the muscles acting on the shoulder complex.[32-39]

The sternoclavicular and acromioclavicular joints contribute to scapulohumeral rhythm by synergistic muscle activity of the serratus anterior and trapezius muscles which produce the necessary upward rotation of the scapula. The first 30 degrees of scapulothoracic motion involve the elevation of the clavicle at the sternoclavicular joint. This elevation of the clavicle swings the scapula through an arc of motion to avoid the ligamentous limitations which are present in the shoulder complex. During the last 30 degrees of scapulothoracic motion, elevation of the sternal end of the clavicle can no longer continue; therefore, the acromioclavicular joint acts to elevate the clavicle at the acromion end, again avoiding ligamentous limitation.[4,5,30,37,40-44]

REACHING FOR AND GRASPING THE RAZOR

At the outset of this activity, the individual was standing in the anatomical position in front of the washstand. As the individual reached to grasp the razor (Figure 2-2), the shoulder joint flexed 10 to 20 degrees, with the prime movers being the anterior deltoid, the coracobrachialis, and the pectoralis major muscles.[37,42] The deltoid muscle acted concentrically to produce an upward translatory motion on the humerus. When the pectoralis major muscle contracted concentrically, the proximoanterior aspect of the humerus was drawn closer to the rib cage, or adduction and inward rotation of the humerus occurred.[29] This muscular component was important to cancel the abduction component of the deltoid without interfering with the flexion component. Concentric contraction of the coracobrachialis muscle drew the proximal part of the humerus closer to the coracoid process, creating almost pure shoulder flexion.[7,9]

Flexion of the elbow complex was also needed for the reaching and grasping component of this activity. The elbow complex moved through approximately 20 to 30 degrees of flexion. Concentric contraction of the biceps brachii, brachialis, and brachioradialis muscles drew the radius and ulna closer to the shoulder complex, as well as drawing the wrist complex closer to the shoulder complex. However, the brachialis muscle alone would have been capable of producing this motion.[45-48]

At the same time that the elbow complex was flexing, the forearm underwent pronation (see Figure 2-2), which occurred at the superior and inferior radioulnar joints.[49] The concentric contraction of the pronator teres and pronator quadratus muscles brought the radioulnar joints into approximately 60 to 70 degrees of pronation, drawing the lateral aspect of the radius closer to the medial aspect of the humerus and pivoting the radius over the ulna.

While the above motions were occurring, simultaneous ulnar deviation of the wrist of approximately 10 degrees was accomplished through the synergistic action of the flexor carpi ulnaris and extensor carpi ulnaris muscles. Wrist extension to 20 to 30 degrees was brought about by concentric activity of the extensors carpi ulnaris, carpi radialis longus, and carpi radialis brevis muscles.[50-52]

Figure 2-2. Reaching for the razor: The shoulder joint has flexed and the forearm has pronated. The key landmarks denoted by black dots are: A = acromion process (dorsal aspect); B = greater tuberosity of humerus; C = lateral epicondyle of humerus; D = ulnar head (dorsal aspect); E = radial styloid process (dorsal aspect); H = ulnar styloid process (ulnar aspect); and I = fifth MCP joint line (ulnar aspect).

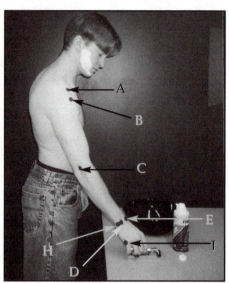

As the individual began to grasp the razor, a pad-to-pad, three-jaw chuck grip was used to facilitate precision handling of the razor (Figure 2-3). The MCP and proximal interphalangeal (PIP) joints of digits two and three were partially flexed. The second and third MCP joints flexed 40 and 30 degrees, respectively, while the second and third PIP joints flexed 40 and 55 degrees, respectively. In addition, the distal interphalangeal (DIP) joints of these two digits flexed 20 degrees each. The MCP joint of the thumb flexed 30 to 35 degrees. Minimal or no flexion of the IP joint of the thumb was needed at this time.[53-54]

The prime movers of the MCP joints of digits two and three were the lumbricals and dorsal and palmar interossei muscles, contracting concentrically.[55-57] The prime movers for the PIP and DIP joints were the flexor digitorum superficialis and flexor digitorum profundus muscles, contracting concentrically. The activity of the palmar interossei muscles also caused adduction to occur, which is a component motion of a three-jaw chuck grip.

Concentric contraction of the flexor pollicis longus drew the palmar side of the thumb closer to the anterior aspect of the radius, while concentric contraction of the flexor pollicis brevis drew the anterior aspect of the thumb closer to the anterior aspect of the wrist joint. Concentric contraction of the opponens pollicis muscle brought the thumb in opposition to digits two and three, completing the three-jaw chuck grip.[58]

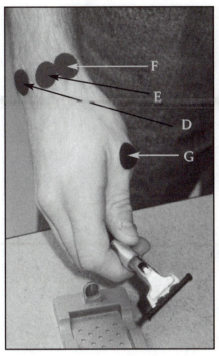

Figure 2-3. Grasping the razor: A pad-to-pad, three-jaw chuck was used. The key landmarks denoted by black dots are: D = ulnar head (dorsal aspect); E = radial styloid process (dorsal aspect); F = radial styloid process (radial aspect); and G = first MCP joint line (radial aspect).

BRINGING THE RAZOR TO THE FACE

Now that the individual had reached for and grasped the razor, the razor had to be brought to the face. First, the superior and inferior radioulnar joints were supinated to the neutral position (Figure 2-4). This action was brought about by the concentric contraction of the biceps brachii and supinator muscles. As these muscles contracted, the radius was brought back over the ulna, bringing the radius closer to the lateral side of the distal humerus.

Simultaneously, the elbow joint was flexed from its 20 to 30 degree position to 130 to 140 degrees, while the shoulder joint was flexed from its 10 to 20 degree position to 40 to 50 degrees and was abducted to 30 to 40 degrees (see Figure 2-4). During this entire activity, the hand maintained the three-jaw chuck grip.[59] The concentric activity of the biceps brachii that brought the elbow joint into this position also enabled this muscle to supinate the forearm.[48]

The shoulder joint muscles described in the first part of this activity continued to cause further flexion of the joint. There was an added abduction component brought about by the middle fibers of the deltoid

Figure 2-4. Bringing the razor to the face: The shoulder and elbow joints were flexed and the forearm was supinated. The key landmarks denoted by black dots are: A = acromion process (dorsal aspect); B = greater tuberosity of humerus; C = lateral epicondyle of humerus; D = ulnar head (dorsal aspect); E = radial styloid process (dorsal aspect); and H = ulnar styloid process (ulnar aspect).

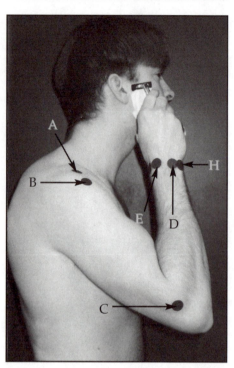

muscle, acting concentrically.[28, 60-62] The three-jaw chuck grip was maintained by isometric activity of the hand muscles previously described.

PERFORMING THE STROKING MOTIONS

To complete the task of shaving, the individual began to perform the third step in this activity: executing the downward and upward strokes of the razor on the face (Figures 2-5 and 2-6). The stroke included shoulder flexion, extension, abduction, and adduction. The elbow joint remained flexed to 140 degrees, and the forearm was maintained in the neutral position (see Figure 2-6), while the three-jaw chuck grip was sustained (Figure 2-7).

The latissimus dorsi, teres major, and posterior deltoid muscles were involved in controlling shoulder extension, which helped to complete the downward stroke of the razor.[63] Since control was needed, the powerful concentric actions of these muscles were overridden by the eccentric activity of the shoulder flexor muscles which have been described previously. Otherwise, the razor would have been brought too far downward and

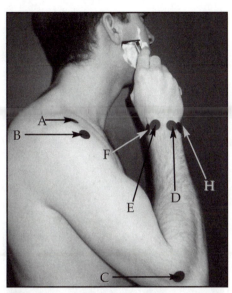

Figure 2-5. Downward stroking motion: The shoulder joint was extended, abducted, and adducted. The key landmarks denoted by black dots are: A = acromion process (dorsal aspect); B = greater tuberosity of humerus; C = lateral epicondyle of humerus; D = ulnar head (dorsal aspect); E = radial styloid process (dorsal aspect); F = radial styloid process (radial aspect); and H = ulnar styloid process (ulnar aspect).

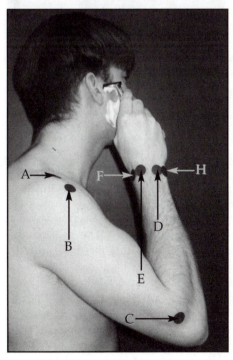

Figure 2-6. Upward stroking motion: The shoulder joint was flexed and abducted. The key landmarks denoted by black dots are: A = acromion process (dorsal aspect); B = greater tuberosity of humerus; C = lateral epicondyle of humerus; D = ulnar head (dorsal aspect); E = radial styloid process (dorsal aspect); F = radial styloid process (radial aspect); and H = ulnar styloid process (ulnar aspect).

Figure 2-7. Hand position during the upward stroking motion: A three-jaw chuck was maintained. The key landmarks denoted by black dots are: D = ulnar head (dorsal aspect); E = radial styloid process (dorsal aspect); F = radial styloid process (radial aspect); and G = first MCP joint line (radial aspect).

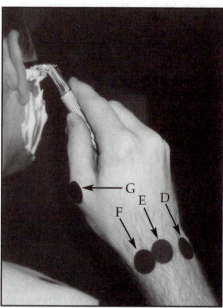

required more muscular activity and joint range than was actually needed to complete the task. The same can be said for the shoulder adduction which occurred during this time. The eccentric activity of the previously described shoulder abductor muscles controlled this movement.

Once the downward stroke had been completed, the process was reversed and the upward stroke of this activity was initiated (see Figure 2-6). The upward stroke involved abduction of the shoulder joint which has been described previously. The remainder of this third step of the process was a repetition of downward and upward strokes until the face had been shaved completely.[64-65]

There is a need, however, to discuss the differences seen in shaving the ipsilateral and the contralateral sides of the face. The primary differences were in the amounts of shoulder joint rotation, both internal and external, needed to complete the task.[66-67] As the individual moved to the contralateral side of the face, more internal rotation of the shoulder joint was noted. As the individual completed the shaving of the face and returned the razor to the washstand, more external rotation of the shoulder joint was noted. Although these differences may seem minimal, it is important to be aware of them, as it is not unusual to see limitations in an individual's ability to rotate the shoulder joint following injury to the more proximal part of the upper extremity.[68]

SUMMARY

Key Anatomical Landmarks for Shaving Analysis

Shoulder Complex:	Greater tuberosity of humerus Acromion process (dorsal aspect)
Elbow and Forearm Complex:	Lateral epicondyle of humerus Radial styloid process (dorsal aspect) Radial styloid process (radial aspect) Ulnar head (dorsal aspect) Ulnar styloid process (ulnar aspect)
Wrist and Hand Complex:	Base of first MCP (radial and palmar aspects) Base of second MCP (dorsal aspect) Base of fifth MCP (dorsal aspect) First MCP joint line (palmar aspect) Second MCP joint line (radial aspect) Fifth MCP joint line (ulnar aspect) First IP joint line (palmar aspect) Second PIP joint line (radial aspect) Fifth PIP joint line (ulnar aspect) Second DIP joint line (radial aspect) Fifth DIP joint line (ulnar aspect)

Major Phases for Shaving Analysis

Starting Position

- Position of subject

- Height of counter

- Position of razor

- Type of razor

Reaching For and Grasping the Razor

Bringing the Razor to the Face

Performing the Stroking Motions

- Ipsilateral side of face

- Contralateral side of face

Upper Extremity Joint Motions and Muscular Activity: Shaving the Face

Introduction and Set-Up

- All joints start in the anatomical position.

Reaching For and Grasping the Razor
- Primarily flexion of the proximal and distal joints.

- Pronation of radioulnar joint.

- Ulnar deviation and extension of wrist joint.

- Concentric contractions of flexors, pronators, and wrist extensors.

Bringing the Razor to the Face
- Primarily flexion of proximal joints.

- Supination of radioulnar joint.

- Distal joints maintain positions.

- Concentric contractions of flexors and supinators.

- Isometric contractions of distal muscles.

Performing the Stroking Motions—Downward Stroke
- Primarily flexion and abduction of shoulder joint followed by extension and adduction of shoulder joint.

- Distal joints maintain positions.

- Concentric contractions for shoulder flexors and abductors followed by eccentric contractions.

- Isometric contractions of distal muscles.

Performing the Stroking Motions—Upward Stroke

- Shoulder joint is the same as that described for bringing the razor to the face.

- This is a reversal of the downward stroke.
- All other joints are maintaining positions via isometric muscular contraction.

CLINICAL APPLICATION AND DISCUSSION QUESTIONS

Many male patients/clients include shaving the face as one of their activities of daily living. The ability to perform such an activity can be limited due to various injuries or disabilities, such as rotator cuff tears, lateral epicondylitis, radial nerve palsy, carpal tunnel syndrome, and/or upper extremity paralysis secondary to a cerebral vascular accident. The specific muscles involved in any of these injuries, and the motions that these muscles produce, have an impact on the individual's ability to perform this task.

In some instances, other muscles may be substituted for the involved muscles, thereby enabling the individual to complete the task unassisted. Make a list of the possible muscle substitutions for this activity. Compare your list of substitutions to those in Chart 1 in Appendix A.

In other instances, the use of assistive devices or switching hand dominance may be necessary to enable the individual to function. Any of these changes would result in variations of the manner in which the activity is completed. For instance, compare this analysis to that using an electric razor instead of a standard razor. Would there be a significant difference in the shoulder and elbow joint activity? Would the hand grip used change?

Next, make a list of assistive devices that would be of value in performing this activity. Discuss how each would be of benefit to the person doing the activity.

What other injuries to the shoulder complex, the elbow and forearm complex, or the wrist and hand complex would affect the individual's ability to complete this activity? What other muscle substitutions could be used to complete the activity?

Compare this muscular analysis to that of shaving the legs. What are the significant differences in performing this activity?

Finally, compare this muscular analysis to other activities of daily living that involve the upper trunk and head regions, such as brushing the teeth, brushing the hair, or applying makeup.

Remember, functional outcomes are based on sound clinical problem-solving and reasoning. Knowing the fundamental kinesiological and biomechanical applications will make clinical problem-solving and reasoning easier, more effective, and more efficient.

REFERENCES

1. Bechtol C. Biomechanics of the shoulder. *Clin Orthop.* 1980;146:37-41.
2. Carmichael SW, Hart DL. Anatomy of the shoulder joint. *J Orthop Sports Phys Ther.* 1985;6:225-228.
3. Perry T. Normal upper extremity kinesiology. *Phys Ther.* 1978;58:165-178.
4. Dvir Z, Berme N. The shoulder complex in elevation of the arm: a mechanism approach. *J Biomech.* 1978;11:219-225.
5. Högfors C, Sigholm G, Herberts P. Biomechanical model of the human shoulder. I .Elements. *J Biomech.* 1987;20:157-166.
6. Culham E, Peat M. Functional anatomy of the shoulder complex. *J Orthop Sports Phys Ther.* 1993;18:342-350.
7. Quiring DP, Boroush EL. Functional anatomy of the shoulder girdle. *Arch Phys Med Rehabil.* 1946;27:90-96.
8. Rothman RH, Marvel JP, Heppenstall RB. Anatomic considerations in the glenohumeral joint. *Orthop Clin North Am.* 1975;6:341-352.
9. Schenkman M, DeCartaya VR. Kinesiology of the shoulder complex. *J Orthop Sports Phys Ther.* 1987;8:438-450.
10. Ishizuki M. Functional anatomy of the elbow joint and three-dimensional quantitative analysis of the elbow joint. *Journal of the Japanese Orthopedic Association.* 1979;53:986-989.
11. London JT. Kinematics of the elbow. *J Bone Joint Surg Am.* 1981;63:529-535.
12. Morrey BF, Askew LJ, An KN, Chao EY. A biomechanical study of normal and functional elbow motion. *J Bone Joint Surg Am.* 1981;63:872-877.
13. Stroyan M, Wilk KE. The functional anatomy of the elbow complex. *J Orthop Sports Phys Ther.* 1993;17:279-288.
14. Andrews JG, Youm Y. A biomechanical investigation of wrist kinematics. *J Biomech.* 1979;12:83-93.
15. Brumfield RH, Champoux JA. A biomechanical study of normal functional wrist motion. *Clin Orthop.* 1979;187:23-25.
16. Erdman AG, Mayfield JK, Dorman F, Wallrich M, Dahlof W. Kinematic and kinetic analysis of the human wrist by stereoscopic instrumentation. *J Biomech Eng.* 1979;101:124-133.
17. Kauer JMG. Functional anatomy of the wrist. *Clin Orthop.* 1980;149:9-20.
18. Linscheid RL. Kinematic considerations of the wrist. *Clin Orthop.* 1986;202:27-39.

19. Radonjic D, Long CL. Kinesiology of the wrist. *Am J Phys Med Rehabil.* 1971;50:57-71.

20. Ryu J, Cooney WP, Askew LJ, An KN, Chao EYS. Functional ranges of motion of the wrist joint. *J Hand Surg [Am].* 1991;16:409-419.

21. Volz RG, Lieb M, Benjamin J. Biomechanics of the wrist. *Clin Orthop.* 1980;149:112-117.

22. Wadsworth CT. Clinical anatomy and mechanics of the wrist and hand. *J Orthop Sports Phys Ther.* 1983;4:206-216.

23. An KN, Chao EY, Conney WP, Linscheid RI. Normative model of human hand for biomechanical analysis. *J Biomech.* 1979;12:775-788.

24. Buchholz B, Armstrong TJ. A kinematic model of the human hand to evaluate its prehensile abilities. *J Biomech.* 1992;25:149-162.

25. Craig SM. Anatomy of the joints of the fingers. *Hand Clin.* 1992;8:693-700.

26. Landsmeer JMF. Power grip and precision handling. *Ann Rheum Dis.* 1962;21:164-170.

27. Taylor CL, Schwarz RJ. The anatomy and mechanics of the human hand. *Artificial Limbs.* 1955;2:22-34.

28. Bagg SD, Forrest WJ. A biomechanical analysis of scapular rotation during arm abduction in the scapular plane. *Am J Phys Med Rehabil.* 1988;67:238-245.

29. Blakely RL, Palmer ML. Analysis of rotation accompanying shoulder flexion. *Phys Ther.* 1984;64:1214-1216.

30. Högfors C, Peterson B, Sigholm G, Herberts P. Biomechanical model of the human shoulder joint. II. The shoulder rhythm. *J Biomech.* 1991;24:699-709.

31. Poppen NK, Walker PS. Normal and abnormal motion of the shoulder. *J Bone Joint Surg Am.* 1976;58:195-201.

32. Atkeson CG. Learning arm kinematics and dynamics. *Annu Rev Neurosci.* 1989;12:157-183.

33. Atkeson CG, Hollerbach JM. Kinematic features of unrestrained vertical arm movements. *J Neurosci.* 1985;5:2318-2330.

34. Basset RW, Browne AO, Morrey BF, An KN. Glenohumeral muscle force and moment mechanics in a position of shoulder instability. *J Biomech.* 1990;23:405-412.

35. Engin AE. On the biomechanics of the shoulder complex. *J Biomech.* 1980;13:575-590.

36. Kent BE. Functional anatomy of the shoulder complex: a review. *Phys Ther.* 1971;51:867-888.

37. Kronberg M, Nemeth G, Brostrom L. Muscle activity and coordination in the normal shoulder. *Clin Orthop.* 1990;257:76-85.

38. Peat M. Functional anatomy of the shoulder complex. *Phys Ther.* 1986;66:1855-1865.

39. Saha AK. Dynamic stability of the glenohumeral joint. *Acta Orthop Scand.* 1971;42:491-505.

40. Conway AM. Movements at the sternoclavicular and acromioclavicular joints. *Phys Ther.* 1961;11:421-432.

41. Hart DL, Carmichael SW. Biomechanics of the shoulder. *J Orthop Sports Phys Ther.* 1985;16:229-278.

42. Inman VT, Saunders JB. Observations on the functions of the clavicle. *California Medicine.* 1946;65:158-166.

43. Pearl ML, Perry J, Torburn L, Gordon LH. An electromyographic analysis of the shoulder during cones and planes of arm motion. *Clin Orthop.* 1992;284:116-127.

44. Browne AL, An KN, Tanaka S, Morrey BF. Glenohumeral elevation studied in three dimensions. *J Bone Joint Surg Br.* 1990;72:843-845.

45. An KN, Hui FC, Morrey BF, Linscheid RL, Chao EY. Muscles across the elbow joint: a biomechanical analysis. *J Biomech.* 1981;14:659-669.

46. Basmajian JV, Latif A. Integrated actions and functions of the chief flexors of the elbow: a detailed electromyographic analysis. *J Bone Joint Surg Am.* 1957;39:1106-1118.

47. Pauly JE, Rushing JL, Scheving LE. An electromyographic study of some muscles crossing the elbow joint. *Anat Rec.* 1967;159:47-53.

48. Van Zuylen EJ, Van Velzen A. A biomechanical model for flexion torque of human arm muscles as a function of elbow angle. *J Biomech.* 1988;21:183-189.

49. Ray RD, Johnson RJ, Jameson RM. Rotation of the forearm: an experimental study of pronation and supination. *J Bone Joint Surg Am.* 1951;33:993-996.

50. Sarrafian SK, Melamed JL, Goshgarian GM. Study of wrist motion in flexion and extension. *Clin Orthop.* 1977;126:153-159.

51. Youm Y, McMurty RY, Flatt AE, Gillespie TE. Kinematics of the wrist. I. An experimental study of radial-ulnar deviation and flexion-extension. *J Bone Joint Surg Am.* 1978;60:423-432.

52. Youm Y, Yoon YS. Analytical development in investigation of wrist kinematics. *J Biomech.* 1979;12:613-621.

53. Barmakian JT. Anatomy of the joints of the thumb. *Hand Clin.* 1992;8:683-691.

54. Iameda T, An K, Cooney WP. Functional anatomy and biomechanics of the thumb. *Hand Clin.* 1992;8:9-15.

55. Backhouse KM, Catton WT. An experimental study of the function of the lumbrical muscles in the human hand. *J Anat.* 1954;88:133-137.

56. Leijnse JNAL, Kalker IJ. A two dimensional kinematic model of the lumbrical in the human finger. *J Biomech.* 1995;28:237-249.

57. Youm Y, Gillespie TE, Flatt AE, Sprague BL. Kinematic investigation of normal MCP joint. *J Biomech.* 1978;11:109-118.

58. Long C, Conrad PW, Hall EA, Furler SL. Intrinsic-extrinsic muscle control of the hand in power grip and precision handling: an electromyographic study. J Bone Joint Surg Br. 1970;52:853-867.

59. Chao EY, Opgrande JD, Axmear FE. Three-dimensional force analysis of finger joints in selected isometric hand functions. J Biomech. 1976;9:387-396.

60. Doody SG, Freedman L, Waterland JC. Shoulder movement during abduction in the scapular plane. Arch Phys Med Rehabil. 1970;51.595-604.

61. Freedman L, Munro RR. Abduction of the arm in the scapular plane: scapular and glenohumeral movements. J Bone Joint Surg Am. 1966;48:1503-1510.

62. Walker PS, Poppen NK. Biomechanics of the shoulder joint during abduction in the plane of the scapula. Bull Hosp Jt Dis. 1977;38:107-111.

63. Broome HL, Basmajian JV. The function of the teres major muscle: an electromyographic study. Anat Rec. 1970;170:309-310.

64. Hagberg M. Workload and fatigue in repetitive arm elevations. Ergonomics. 1981;24:543-555.

65. Herberts P, Kadefors R, Broman H. Arm positioning in manual tasks—an electromyographic study of localized muscle fatigue. Ergonomics. 1980;23:655-665.

66. Soderberg GJ, Blaschak MJ. Shoulder internal and external rotation peak torque production. J Orthop Sports Phys Ther. 1987;8:518-524.

67. Walmsley RP, Szybbo C. A comparative study of the torque generated by the shoulder internal and external rotator muscles in different positions and at varying speeds. J Orthop Sports Phys Ther. 1987;9:217-222.

68. Howell SM, Galinat BJ, Renzi AJ. Normal and abnormal mechanics of the glenohumeral joint in the horizontal plane. J Bone Joint Surg Am. 1988;70:227-232.

SUGGESTED READINGS

Ayoub MM, LoPresti P. The determination of an optimum size cylindrical handle by use of electromyography. Ergonomics. 1971;4:503-518.

Buchholz B, Armstrong TJ, Goldstein SA. Anthropometric data for describing the kinematics of the human hand. Ergonomics. 1992;35:261-273.

Cobb T. Aetiology of work-related carpal tunnel syndrome: the role of lumbrical muscles and tool size on carpal tunnel. Ergonomics. 1996;39:103-15.

Cooney WP, Chao EYS. Biomechanical analysis of static forces of the thumb during hand function. J Bone Joint Surg Am. 1977;59:27-36.

DeLuca CJ, Forrest WJ. Force analysis of individual muscles acting simultaneously on the shoulder joint during isometric abduction. J Biomech. 1973;6:385-393.

Engen TJ, Spencer WA. Method of kinematic study of normal upper extremity movements. Arch Phys Med Rehabil. 1968;49:9-11.

Gerdle B, Elert J, Henriksson-Larsen K. Muscular fatigue during repeated iso-kinetic shoulder forward flexions in young females. *Eur J Appl Physiol.* 1988;57:415-419.

Gerdle B, Eriksson NE, Hagberg C. Changes in the surface electromyogram during increasing isometric shoulder forward flexion. *Eur J Appl Physiol.* 1988;57:404-408.

Hagberg C, Hagberg M. Surface EMG amplitude and frequency dependence on exerted force for the upper trapezius muscle: a comparison between right and left sides. *Eur J Appl Physiol.* 1989;58:641-645.

Howell SM, Imoberseg AM, Seger DH, Marone PJ. Clarification of the role of the supraspinatus muscle in shoulder function. *J Bone Joint Surg Am.* 1985;68:398-404.

Hsia PT, Drury CG. A simple method of evaluating handle design. *Appl Ergonomics.* 1986;17:209-213.

Inman VT, Saunders JB, Abbott LC. Observations on the function of the shoulder joint. *J Bone Joint Surg Am.* 1944;26:1-30.

Jarp Y. Activation of the rotator cuff in generating isometric shoulder rotation torque. *Am J Sports Med.* 1996;24:477-485.

Kuhlman JR, Iannotti JP, Kelly MJ, Riegler FX, Gevaert ML, Ergin TM. Isokinetic and isometric measurement of strength of external rotation and abduction of the shoulder. *J Bone Joint Surg Am.* 1992;74:1320-1333.

Lange A, Kauer JMG, Huiskes R. Kinematic behavior of the human wrist joint: a roentgen-stereophotogrammateric analysis. *J Orthop Res.* 1985;3:56-64.

Nemeth G, Kronberg M, Brostrom L. Electromyograph (EMG) recordings from the subscapularis muscle: description of a technique. *J Orthop Res.* 1990;8:151-153.

Otis JC, Warren RF, Backus SI, Santner TJ, Mahey JD. The interaction of function, dominance, joint angle, and angular velocity. Torque production in the shoulder of the normal young adult male. *Am J Sports Med.* 1990;18:119-123.

Tarbet JA, Wolin PM. Rotator cuff. *Phys Sports Med J.* 1997;25:54-74.

Van Woensel W, Arwert H. Effects of external load and abduction angle on EMG level of shoulder muscles during isometric action. *Electromyo Clin Neurophysiol.* 1993;33:185-191.

Veeger HE, Van der Helm FC, Vand der Woude LH, Pronk GM, Rozendal RH. Inertia and muscle contraction parameters for musculoskeletal modeling of the shoulder mechanism. *J Biomech.* 1991;24:615-629.

Yoon YS. Analytical development in investigation of wrist kinematics. *J Biomech.* 1979;12:613-621.

Chapter 3

Brushing the Hair

INTRODUCTION AND SET-UP

Brushing the hair can be done in many different ways and at many different locations. For this analysis, the subject was standing in front of a mirror attached to a cabinet. The roll-like brush was on a table, positioned 6 inches from the edge. The table was 2 ½ feet high. The brush had a slender, cylindrical handle. The subject's hair was collar length (Figure 3-1).

Although individuals brush their hair in a variety of methods, emphasis was placed on the technique wherein the upper extremity that was grasping the brush did all the work. Motions at each joint involved in this activity of daily living were analyzed. As mentioned above, the subject was standing in front of the mirror in a modified anatomical position. Therefore, the subject's shoulder joint was in neutral, and the elbow joint was flexed 40 degrees. The hand was held in its natural "resting attitude."[1-2] In other words, the upper extremity was hanging down by the subject's side.

REACHING FOR AND GRASPING THE BRUSH

As the subject reached for the brush, the shoulder joint flexed approximately 45 degrees (Figure 3-2). The anterior fibers of the deltoid, the clavicular fibers of the pectoralis major, and the coracobrachialis muscles were concentrically contracting as the prime movers.[3] In addition, the short head of the biceps brachii and the subscapularis muscles contracted concentrically to assist these prime movers.[4] The subscapularis served an important stabilization role during this time.[5-7] The elbow joint extended 40 degrees during this time, while the radioulnar joint began to pronate approximately 23 degrees.

Figure 3-1. Starting position: Subject standing in front of the table with the brush positioned 6 inches from the edge. The key landmarks denoted by black dots are: A = acromion process (dorsal aspect); B = greater tuberosity of humerus; C = lateral epicondyle; D = ulnar head (dorsal aspect); E = radial styloid process (dorsal aspect); F = radial styloid process (radial aspect); and G = first MCP joint line (radial aspect).

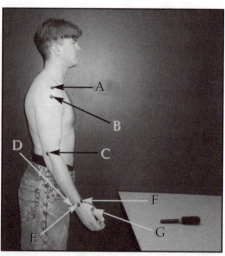

Figure 3-2. Reaching for the brush: The elbow joint was flexed; the elbow joint, extended; and the forearm, pronated. The key landmarks denoted by black dots are: A = acromion process (dorsal aspect); B = greater tuberosity of humerus; C = lateral epicondyle; D = ulnar head (dorsal aspect); E = radial styloid process (dorsal aspect); and I = fifth MCP joint line (ulnar aspect).

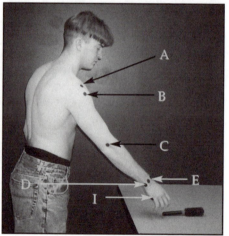

The triceps brachii muscle contracted concentrically to position the elbow joint. Concentric contractions of the pronator teres and the pronator quadratus muscles allowed the wrist motion to occur.[8] At the same time, the subject's wrist joint extended 5 degrees and ulnarly deviated 5 degrees in preparation for grasping the brush.[9-10] The extensors carpi radialii longus and brevis and carpi ulnaris muscles concentrically contracted to accomplish this activity. However, there was a greater effort by the extensor carpi ulnaris muscles to effect the ulnar deviation that was needed.[11] As soon as the wrist was positioned, the muscle activity switched to an isometric contraction to maintain the wrist in the extended position.

Finally, the hand grasped the brush (Figure 3-3). The MCP joints, primarily through concentric contractions of the lumbricals, flexor digitorum superficialis, flexor digiti minimi, opponens digiti minimi, and flexors pollicis longus and brevis muscles, flexed 45 degrees.[12-15] The flexor digitorum profundus and the dorsal and palmar interossei muscles assisted this motion. The PIP joints flexed 30 degrees via concentric contraction of the flexor digitorum superficialis muscle. The DIP joints flexed 1 to 3 degrees through a concentric contraction of the flexor digitorum profundus muscle. The thumb was abducted 1 to 3 degrees by a concentric contraction of the abductor pollicis longus and brevis muscles.[16] All these movements placed the hand in a functional position for grasping.[17-19] The hand, utilizing pad-to-pad prehension, remained in this position to allow the brush to be picked up with minimal flexion of the MCP and PIP joints. The pad of the thumb was positioned on one side of the handle of the brush, while the pads of digits two through five were on the other side of the handle. To maintain this grasp, the lumbricals and the flexor digitorum superficialis muscles were contracting concentrically. The thumb was held in opposition through the concentric contraction of the opponens pollicis muscle.[20]

How to describe the grip once the brush had been grasped? At first, it appeared that a precision grip was being used, which was probably the case. However, once the brush had been grasped, the grip changed to a power grip for the rest of the activity (Figure 3-4).

Most subjects use a cylindrical power grip for the remainder of the activity.[18] This should make sense as the power to brush the hair primarily comes from the shoulder complex with some assistance from the elbow and more distal joint complexes. The greater the thickness and consistency of the hair, the greater the power required to move the brush through the hair.

Figure 3-3. Grasping the brush: The digits were flexed to grasp the brush. The key landmarks denoted by black dots are: A = acromion process (dorsal aspect); B = greater tuberosity of humerus; C = lateral epicondyle; D = ulnar head (dorsal aspect); E = radial styloid process (dorsal aspect); H = ulnar styloid process (ulnar aspect); and I = fifth MCP joint line (ulnar aspect).

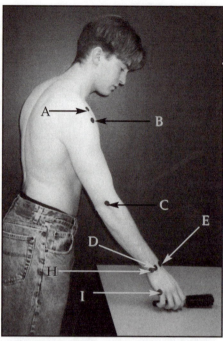

Figure 3-4. Grasping the brush: Close-up cylindrical power grip used to maintain the grasp on the brush throughout the remainder of this activity. The key landmarks denoted by the black dots are: D = ulnar head (dorsal aspect); E = radial styloid process (dorsal aspect); and H = ulnar styloid process (ulnar aspect).

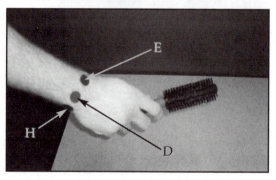

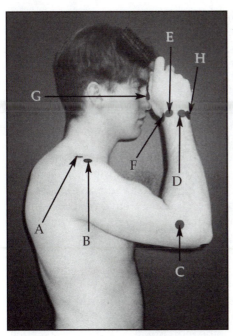

Figure 3-5. Bringing the brush to the top of the head: The shoulder and elbow joints were flexed. The key landmarks denoted by the black dots are: A = acromion process (dorsal aspect); B = greater tuberosity of humerus; C = lateral epicondyle; D = ulnar head (dorsal aspect); E = radial styloid process (dorsal aspect); F = radial styloid process (radial aspect); G = first MCP joint line (radial aspect); and H = ulnar styloid process (ulnar aspect).

BRINGING THE BRUSH TO THE TOP OF THE HEAD

Next, the subject brought the brush to the top of the head (Figure 3-5). To do this, the subject's shoulder joint flexed from 45 to 90 degrees. In addition to the shoulder muscles already cited, concentric activity of the serratus anterior and the upper trapezius muscles contributed to this part of the movement. These two muscles acted synergistically to produce upward rotation of the scapula along the thoracic cage. There was also a contribution from the levator scapulae and rhomboid muscles to help elevate the scapula.[3,4,21-26]

The elbow joint flexed 95 degrees during this time. The muscle activity required for this elbow motion was dependent on the timing of the subject's flexion. If the elbow was flexed prior to the shoulder's second stage of flexion (45 to 90 degrees), a concentric contraction of the biceps brachii muscle accomplished the flexion. However, if the subject flexed the elbow after the shoulder's second stage of flexion, an eccentric contraction of the triceps brachii muscle occurred. Why? In the former movement, gravity needed to be overcome, whereas in the latter movement, gravity needed to be controlled as it was exerting a downward pull on the extremity.[27-32]

During this entire time, the wrist joint and hand remained in the same position since grasping the brush. Up until this time, the more proximal joints had been positioning the wrist and hand for the start of the downward stroke of the brush through the hair on the subject's ipsilateral side.

STROKING MOTIONS DURING BRUSHING

During the downward stroke, the shoulder complex was being depressed (Figure 3-6). The shoulder joint was extending approximately 10 degrees. Gravity was the primary force acting on the subject's upper extremity, while the hair texture provided additional resistance. The inferior fibers of the trapezius muscle may have contracted concentrically to aid in drawing the scapula downward and inward. The rhomboid muscles acted synergistically with the lower trapezius muscle to accomplish this motion.[33]

The elbow joint flexed an additional 20 degrees, moving from 95 to 115 degrees. The elbow flexors, primarily the biceps brachii muscle, concentrically contracted during this time. The radioulnar joint remained in the midposition. (However, please note that this varies from one individual to another. Some individuals will pronate as much as 25 degrees during this time.)

The wrist joint was radially deviating 20 degrees during the downward stroke. A concentric contraction of the flexor and extensor carpi radialii muscles accomplished this movement. The hand grasp remained the same.

To complete brushing the ipsilateral side of the head, the subject returned the upper extremity to the top of the head as each downward stroke was completed. This meant that the subject's upper extremity returned to the starting position by flexing the shoulder joint as previously described (Figure 3-7). The elbow joint was extended back to 95 degrees through a concentric contraction of the triceps brachii muscle,[27-34] and the wrist joint was returned to its starting position at the top of the head.

As the subject proceeded and moved toward the back of the head, there were some differences in movement of the upper extremity and in the muscle activity to accomplish that movement. To reach the back of the head, the subject maintained shoulder flexion through isometric contractions of the muscles previously cited.[3] The subject also horizontally abducted the shoulder joint by using a concentric contraction of the posterior deltoid muscle (Figure 3-8). The middle deltoid muscle helped to maintain the horizontal position.[4,7,35] On the downward stroke, the shoulder joint externally rotated approximately 80 degrees.

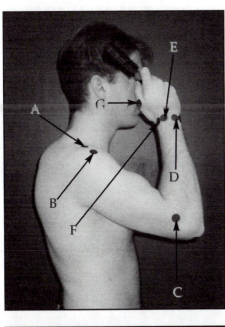

Figure 3-6. Downward stroke during brushing: The shoulder joint depressed; the elbow joint, flexed; and the wrist joint, radially deviated. The key landmarks denoted by black dots are: A = acromion process (dorsal aspect); B = greater tuberosity of humerus; C = lateral epicondyle; D = ulnar head (dorsal aspect); E = radial styloid process (dorsal aspect); F = radial styloid process (radial aspect); and G = first MCP joint line (radial aspect).

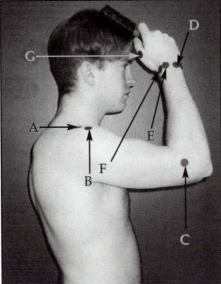

Figure 3-7. Upward stroke to complete brushing the ipsilateral side of the head. The key landmarks denoted by black dots are: A = acromion process (dorsal aspect); B = greater tuberosity of humerus; C = lateral epicondyle; D = ulnar head (dorsal aspect); E = radial styloid process (dorsal aspect); F = radial styloid process (radial aspect); and G = first MCP joint line (radial aspect).

Figure 3-8. Brushing the back of the head: The shoulder joint was horizontally abducted and externally rotated. The key landmarks denoted by black dots are: C = lateral epicondyle; D = ulnar head (dorsal aspect); E = radial styloid process (dorsal aspect); H = ulnar styloid process (ulnar aspect); I = fifth MCP joint line (ulnar aspect); and J = olecranon process.

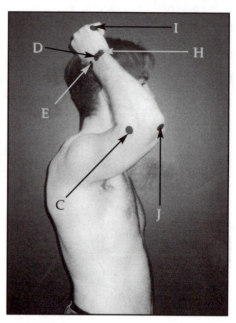

This was accomplished by the infraspinatus and teres minor muscles contracting concentrically.[36-39] The other joints (elbow, radioulnar, and wrist) followed the same pattern of activity as previously described for the ipsilateral side of the head.

To return to the starting position on the back of the head, the shoulder joint moved upward as previously described. However, internal rotation of approximately 80 degrees occurred. Concentric contraction of the internal rotators of the shoulder joint produced this motion, which occurred against gravity. The subscapularis, pectoralis major, latissimus dorsi, and teres major muscles contributed to this activity.[38-39]

BRUSHING THE CONTRALATERAL SIDE OF THE HEAD

Once the entire ipsilateral side and back of the head had been brushed, the subject switched to the contralateral side of the head. This stage of the activity involved horizontal adduction of the shoulder joint, supination of the radioulnar joint, and reversed radial and ulnar deviation of the wrist joint during the stroking motions (Figure 3-9).

The shoulder joint horizontally adducted approximately 45 to 50 degrees. The pectoralis major muscle was the primary mover for shoulder

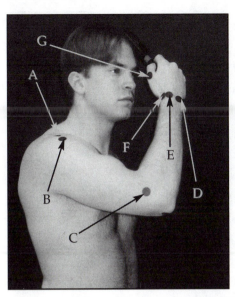

Figure 3-9. Brushing the contralateral side of the head: The shoulder joint was horizontally adducted and internally rotated to reach the top of the head. The key landmarks denoted by the black dots are. A = acromion process (dorsal aspect); B = greater tuberosity of humerus; C = lateral epicondyle; D = ulnar head (dorsal aspect); E = radial styloid process (dorsal aspect); F = radial styloid process (radial aspect); and G = first MCP joint line (radial aspect).

horizontal adduction. A concentric contraction of this muscle enabled the subject to position the upper extremity on the contralateral side of the head. The middle and anterior deltoid muscles acted as stabilizers at this time.[4,26,33,40] In addition, the shoulder joint medially rotated approximately 35 to 40 degrees. Due to the influence of gravity during this time, medial rotation was accomplished through eccentric activity of the lateral rotators of the shoulder joint. The radioulnar joint supinated 30 to 40 degrees through a concentric contraction of the biceps brachii and the supinator muscles.[8] The wrist joint ulnarly deviated to its full extent through concentric contractions of the flexor and extensor carpi ulnaris muscles, with the extensor component contributing a greater effort than the flexor component due to the downward pull of gravity on the wrist joint.[9-11]

During the downward stroke, the same activities as previously reported for the ipsilateral side of the head were repeated at the shoulder and elbow joints. The wrist joint radially deviated 10 degrees past neutral when repositioning the brush at the top of the head. As the subject moved backward on the contralateral side of the head, the activity remained essentially the same. The main difference was in the amount of shoulder horizontal adduction, which increased until it reached its maximum amount at the most posterior aspect of the contralateral side of the head.

SUMMARY

Key Anatomical Landmarks for Brushing Analysis

Shoulder Complex: Greater tuberosity of humerus
                     Acromion process (dorsal aspect)

Elbow and Forearm   Lateral epicondyle of humerus
Complex: Olecranon process
                     Radial styloid process (dorsal aspect)
                     Radial styloid process (radial aspect)
                     Ulnar head (dorsal aspect)
                     Ulnar styloid process (ulnar aspect)

Wrist and Hand   Base of first MCP (radial and palmar aspects)
Complex: Base of second MCP (dorsal aspect)
                     Base of fifth MCP (dorsal aspect)
                     First MCP joint line (palmar aspect)
                     Second MCP joint line (radial aspect)
                     Fifth MCP joint line (ulnar aspect)
                     First IP joint line (palmar aspect)
                     Second PIP joint line (radial aspect)
                     Fifth PIP joint line (ulnar aspect)
                     Second DIP joint line (radial aspect)
                     Fifth DIP joint line (ulnar aspect)

Major Phases for Brushing Analysis
Starting Position
- Position of subject
- Height of dresser
- Position of brush
- Type of brush

Reaching for and Grasping the Brush
Bringing the Brush to the Top of the Head

Stroking Motions During Brushing
- Ipsilateral side of head

- Back of head

Brushing the Contralateral Side of the Head

Upper Extremity Joint Motions and Muscular Activity: Brushing the Hair

Introduction and Set-Up
- The shoulder, radioulnar, and wrist joints start in the anatomical position.

- The thumb and digits 2 through 5 start in the resting attitude.

Reaching for and Grasping the Brush
- Primarily flexion of the proximal and distal joints.

- Extension of the elbow and wrist joints.

- Pronation of the radioulnar joint.

- Ulnar deviation of the wrist joint.

- Abduction and opposition of the thumb CMC joint.

- Concentric contractions of all muscles.

- Isometric contraction of opponens pollicis.

Bringing the Brush to the Top of the Head
- Flexion of shoulder and elbow joints via concentric muscular contraction.

- All other joints are maintaining positions via isometric muscular contraction.

Stroking Motions During Brushing—Downward Stroke—Ipsilateral Side of Head

- Extension of shoulder, with flexion of elbow and radial deviation of wrist joint.

- Primarily concentric muscular contractions.

- All other joints are maintaining positions via isometric muscular contractions.

Stroking Motions During Brushing—Upward Stroke—Ipsilateral Side of Head

- Activity of shoulder, elbow, and wrist joints is the same as that described for bringing the brush to the top of the head (a reversal of the downward stroke).

- All other joints are maintaining their previous positions via isometric muscular activity.

Stroking Motions During Brushing—Upward Stroke—Back of Head

- Shoulder maintains flexed position while internally rotating.

- Concentric muscular activity of internal rotators.

- All other joints followed the same pattern of activity as previously described for the ipsilateral side of the head.

Stroking Motions During Brushing—Downward Stroke—Back of Head

- Extension, horizontal abduction, and external rotation of shoulder joint.

- Concentric muscular activity of horizontal abductors and external rotators.

- All other joints followed the same pattern of activity as previously described for the ipsilateral side of the head.

Brushing the Contralateral Side of the Head—Upward Stroke

• Horizontal adduction and medial rotation of shoulder joint.

• Supination of radioulnar joint.

• Ulnar deviation of wrist joint.

• Primarily concentric contractions of involved muscles.

Brushing the Contralateral Side of the Head— Downward Stroke

• Activity of shoulder, elbow, and wrist joints is the same as that described for the ipsilateral side of the head.

• All other joints are maintaining their previous positions via isometric muscular activity.

CLINICAL APPLICATION AND DISCUSSION QUESTIONS

It should be noted that some individuals switch the brush from one hand to another to brush the two sides of the head. It should also be noted that the type of brush used may alter the hand grip utilized in the activity.[17-18,41-42] The reader is asked to consider how the hand grip would change if a larger handled brush was used instead of the slim-line cylindrical handle used in this analysis. How would the hand grip change with the use of a comb?

For those individuals with more proximal upper extremity problems, fatigue may be a factor in the performance of this activity.[43-46] For others, bursitis[47] or carpal tunnel syndrome[48] may be a factor in performing the activity. Limited range of motion can have an adverse effect on tendon excursion and the length-tension relationship of muscles at a given joint.[20,49-50] In instances of disease or injury, other muscles may substitute for the prime movers.

Make a list of the primary muscles utilized in this activity. Then make a list of muscles that could substitute for the prime movers. Compare your list to Chart 1 in Appendix A.

What other assistive devices might be used to compensate for loss of hand function in an activity such as this? Are there any compensatory motions that could be used elsewhere in the body to compensate for deficits in the upper extremity?

Compare this muscular analysis to the analysis in the previous chapter. How is it similar? How is it different? Observe men and women brushing their hair. Do they use the same technique? If not, how do techniques vary? How does the length of the hair change the analysis? How does the texture of the hair change the analysis?

Finally, compare this analysis to an analysis of brushing a dog's hair. How does the activity change? Is the shoulder joint used the same way? Is the hand grip the same?

REFERENCES

1. Engen TJ, Spencer WA. Method of kinematic study of normal upper extremity movements. *Arch Phys Med Rehabil.* 1968;49:9-11.
2. Perry T. Normal upper extremity kinesiology. *Phys Ther.* 1978;58:165-178.
3. Gerdle B, Eriksson NE, Hagberg C. Changes in the surface electromyogram during increasing isometric shoulder forward flexion. *Eur J Appl Physiol.* 1988;57:404-408.
4. Kronberg M, Nemeth G, Brostrom L. Muscle activity and coordination in the normal shoulder. *Clin Orthop.* 1990;257:76-85.
5. Basset RW, Browne AO, Morrey BF, An KN. Glenohumeral muscle force and moment mechanics in a position of shoulder instability. *J Biomech.* 1990;23:405-412.
6. Nemeth G, Kronberg M, Brostrom L. Electromyogram (EMG) recordings from the subscapularis muscle: description of a technique. *J Orthop Res.* 1990;8:151-153.
7. Saha AK. Dynamic stability of the glenohumeral joint. *Acta Orthop Scand.* 1971;42:491-505.
8. Ray RD, Johnson RJ, Jameson RM. Rotation of the forearm: an experimental study of pronation and supination. *J Bone Joint Surg Am.* 1951;33:993-996.
9. Ryu J, Cooney WP, Askew LJ, An KN, Chao EYS. Functional ranges of motion of the wrist joint. *J Hand Surg [Am].* 1991;16:409-419.
10. Youm Y, McMurty RY, Flatt AE, Gillespie TE. Kinematics of the wrist. I. An experimental study of radial-ulnar deviation and flexion-extension. *J Bone Joint Surg Am.* 1978;60:423-432.
11. Kauer JMG. Functional anatomy of the wrist. *Clin Orthop.* 1980;149:9-20.
12. Backhouse KM, Catton WT. An experimental study of the function of the lumbrical muscles in the human hand. *J Anat.* 1954;88:133-137.
13. Brand PW, Cranor KC, Ellis JC. Tendon and pulleys at the metacarpophalangeal joint of a finger. *J Bone Joint Surg Am.* 1975;57:779-784.
14. Leijnse JNAL, Kalker IJ. A two-dimensional kinematic model of the lumbrical in the human finger. *J Biomech.* 1995;28:237-249.

15. Long C, Conrad PW, Hall EA, Furler SL. Intrinsic-extrinsic muscle control of the hand in power grip and precision handling: an electromyographic study. *J Bone Joint Surg Br.* 1970;52:853-867.

16. Iameda T, An K, Cooney WP. Functional anatomy and biomechanics of the thumb. *Hand Clin.* 1992;8:9-15.

17. Buchholz B, Armstrong TJ. A kinematic model of the human hand to evaluate its prehensile abilities. *J Biomech.* 1992;25:149-162.

18. Landsmeer JMF. Power grip and precision handling. *Ann Rheum Dis.* 1962;21:164-170.

19. Taylor CL, Schwarz RJ. The anatomy and mechanics of the human hand. *Artificial Limbs.* 1955;2:22-34.

20. Jones LA. The assessment of hand function: a critical review of techniques. *J Hand Surg Am.* 1989;14:221-228.

21. An KN, Browne AO, Tanaka S, Morrey BF. Three-dimensional kinematics of glenohumeral elevation. *J Orthop Res.* 1991;9:143-149.

22. Atkeson CG, Hollerbach JM. Kinematic features of unrestrained vertical arm movements. *J Neurosci.* 1985;5:2318-2330.

23. Bechtol C. Biomechanics of the shoulder. *Clin Orthop.* 1980;146:37-41.

24. Browne AO, An KN, Tanaka S, Morrey BF. Glenohumeral elevation studied in three dimensions. *J Bone Joint Surg Br.* 1990;72:843-845.

25. Hagberg C, Hagberg M. Surface EMG amplitude and frequency dependence on exerted force for the upper trapezius muscle: a comparison between right and left sides. *Eur J Appl Physiol.* 1989;58:641-645.

26. Quiring DP, Boroush EL. Functional anatomy of the shoulder girdle. *Arch Phys Med Rehabil.* 1946;27:90-96.

27. An KN, Hui FC, Morrey BF, Linscheid RL, Chao EY. Muscles across the elbow joint: a biomechanical analysis. *J Biomech.* 1981;14:659-669.

28. Basmajian JV, Latif A. Integrated actions and functions of the chief flexors of the elbow: a detailed electromyographic analysis. *J Bone Joint Surg Am.* 1957;39:1106-1118.

29. Shizuki M. Functional anatomy of the elbow joint and three-dimensional quantitative analysis of the elbow joint. *Journal of the Japanese Orthopedic Association.* 1979;53:986-989.

30. Ober AG. An electromyographic analysis of elbow flexors during submaximal concentric contractions. *Res Q Exerc Sport.* 1988;59:139-143.

31. Pauly JE, Rushing JL, Scheving LE. An electromyographic study of some muscles crossing the elbow joint. *Anat Rec.* 1967;159:47-53.

32. Van Zuylen EJ, Van Velzen A. A biomechanical model for flexion torque of human arm muscles as a function of elbow angle. *J Biomech.* 1988;21:183-189.

33. Kent BE. Functional anatomy of the shoulder complex: a review. *Phys Ther.* 1971;51:867-888.

34. Little AD, Lehmkuhl D. Elbow extension force measured in three positions. *Phys Ther*. 1966;46:7-17.

35. Howell SM, Galinat BJ, Renzi AJ. Normal and abnormal mechanics of the glenohumeral joint in the horizontal plane. *J Bone Joint Surg Am*. 1988;70:227-232.

36. Jarp Y. Activation of the rotator cuff in generating isometric shoulder rotation torque. *Am J Sports Med*. 1996;24:477-485.

37. Kuhlman JR, Iannotti JP, Kelly MJ, Riegler FX, Gevaert ML, Ergin TM. Isokinetic and isometric measurement of strength of external rotation and abduction of the shoulder. *J Bone Joint Surg Am*. 1992;74:1320-1333.

38. Soderberg GJ, Blaschak MJ. Shoulder internal and external rotation peak torque production. *J Orthop Sports Phys Ther*. 1987;8:518-524.

39. Walmsley RP, Szybbo C. A comparative study of the torque generated by the shoulder internal and external rotator muscles in different positions and at varying speeds. *J Orthop Sports Phys Ther*. 1987;9:217-222.

40. Högfors C, Sigholm G, Herberts P. Biomechanical model of the human shoulder. I. Elements. *J Biomech*. 1987;20:157-166.

41. Ayoub MM, LoPresti P. The determination of an optimum size cylindrical handle by use of electromyography. *Ergonomics*. 1971;4:503-518.

42. Hsia PT, Drury CG. A simple method of evaluating handle design. *Appl Ergonomics*. 1986;17:209-213.

43. Gerdle B, Elert J, Henriksson-Larsen K. Muscular fatigue during repeated isokinetic shoulder forward flexions in young females. *Eur J Appl Physiol*. 1988;57:415-419.

44. Hagberg M. Workload and fatigue in repetitive arm elevations. *Ergonomics*. 1981;24:543-555.

45. Hagberg M. Electromyographic signs of shoulder muscular fatigue in two elevated arm positions. *Am J Phys Med Rehabil*. 1981;60:111-121.

46. Herberts P, Kadefors R, Broman H. Arm positioning in manual tasks—an electromyographic study of localized muscle fatigue. *Ergonomics*. 1980;23:655-665.

47. Salzman KL. Upper extremity bursitis. *Am Fam Physician*. 1997;56:1797-1812.

48. Cobb T. Aetiology of work-related carpal tunnel syndrome: the role of lumbrical muscles and tool size on carpal tunnel. *Ergonomics*. 1996;39:103-105.

49. An KN, Chao EY, Cooney WP, Linscheid RI. Tendon excursion and moment arm of index finger muscles. *J Biomech*. 1983;16:419-426.

50. Minamikawa Y, Horii E, Amadio PC, Cooney WP, Linscheid RL, An KN. Stability and constraint of the proximal interphalangeal joint. *J Hand Surg Am*. 1993;18:198-204.

SUGGESTED READINGS

An KN, Chao EY, Cooney WP, Linscheid RI. Normative model of human hand for biomechanical analysis. *J Biomech.* 1979;12:775-788.

Brumfield RH, Champoux JA. A biomechanical study of normal functional wrist motion. *Clin Orthop.* 1979;187:23-25.

Carmichael SW, Hart DL. Anatomy of the shoulder joint. *J Orthop Sports Phys Ther.* 1985;6:225-228.

Culham E, Peat M. Functional anatomy of the shoulder complex. *J Orthop Sports Phys Ther.* 1993;18:342-350.

Currier DP. Maximal isometric tension of the elbow extensors at varied positions. *Phys Ther.* 1972;52:1043-1049.

Dvir Z, Berme N. The shoulder complex in elevation of the arm: a mechanism approach. *J Biomech.* 1978;11:219-225.

Engin AE. On the biomechanics of the shoulder complex. *J Biomech.* 1980;13:575 590.

Hart DL, Carmicheal SW. Biomechanics of the shoulder. *J Orthop Sports Phys Ther.* 1985;16:229-278.

London JT. Kinematics of the elbow. *J Bone Joint Surg Am.* 1981;63:529-535.

Morrey BF, Askew LJ, An KN, Chao EY. A biomechanical study of normal and functional elbow motion. *J Bone Joint Surg Am.* 1981;63:872-877.

Peat M. Functional anatomy of the shoulder complex. *Phys Ther.* 1986;66:1855-1865.

Poppen NK, Walker PS. Normal and abnormal motion of the shoulder. *J Bone Joint Surg Am.* 1976;58:195-201.

Radonjic D, Long CL. Kinesiology of the wrist. *Am J Phys Med Rehabil.* 1971;50:57-71.

Schenkman M, DeCartaya VR. Kinesiology of the shoulder complex. *J Orthop Sports Phys Ther.* 1987;8:438-450.

Stroyan M, Wilk KE. The functional anatomy of the elbow complex. *J Orthop Sports Phys Ther.* 1993;17:279-288.

Van Woensel W, Arwert H. Effects of external load and abduction angle on EMG level of shoulder muscles during isometric action. *Electromyogr Clin Neurophysiol.* 1993;33:185-191.

Volz RG, Lieb M, Benjamin J. Biomechanics of the wrist. *Clin Orthop.* 1980;149:112-117.

Wadsworth CT. Clinical anatomy and mechanics of the wrist and hand. *J Orthop Sports Phys Ther.* 1983;4:206-216.

Chapter 4

Donning and Buttoning a Shirt

INTRODUCTION AND SET-UP

When donning a shirt, the need for hand dexterity becomes evident as an individual starts to button the shirt. Given that there are male- and female-tailored shirts, this analysis was limited to a male-tailored shirt; ie, one with buttons on the right and buttonholes on the left as the shirt is in place on the subject's torso, with the buttonholes running vertically and numbering five in total. In this particular analysis, the subject, starting at the first button, buttoned from top to bottom.

REMOVING THE SHIRT FROM A HANGER

To start the analysis, the subject removed the unbuttoned shirt from a hanger at a height of 72 inches, with the subject approximately 30 inches from the hanger (Figure 4-1). The right shoulder and elbow joints flexed to accomplish this task. At the same time, there was a combination of wrist extension, ulnar deviation, and flexion, extension, and abduction of the hand complex to grasp the shirt. The shoulder joint moved from the neutral or rest position to 94 degrees of flexion and then returned to the starting position. The elbow and forearm complex started at neutral as well. The elbow joint flexed 10 degrees, while the forearm remained in a neutral position the entire time. The wrist joint moved from neutral to 11 degrees of flexion and 21 degrees of ulnar deviation.

The movements of the digits varied as the analysis proceeded from thumb to fifth digit. The thumb CMC joint moved from neutral to 18 degrees of abduction and remained the same to complete this task. The thumb MCP joint moved from neutral to 33 degrees of flexion as the shirt was grasped. The thumb IP joint moved from neutral to 30 degrees

Figure 4-1. Starting position: Reaching for the shirt. The key landmarks denoted by black dots are: B = greater tuberosity of humerus; C = lateral epicondyle of humerus; D = ulnar head (dorsal aspect); E = radial styloid process (dorsal aspect); H = ulnar styloid process (ulnar aspect); and I = fifth MCP joint line (ulnar aspect).

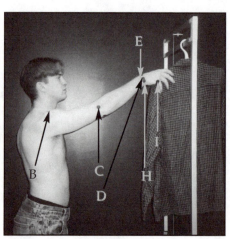

of flexion to complete the task. The second digit started in neutral at the MCP, PIP, and DIP joints. The MCP moved to 3 degrees of hyperextension and then returned to 60 degrees of flexion, the PIP joint moved to 79 degrees of flexion, and the DIP joint moved to 60 degrees of flexion (Figure 4-2).

All the joints of the third through fifth digits also started in neutral. The MCP of the third digit moved to 2 degrees of extension, returned to 74 degrees of flexion, and then abducted 6 degrees. The PIP joint moved to 78 degrees of flexion, and the DIP joint, to 58 degrees of flexion. The fourth digit MCP joint moved to 79 degrees of flexion, abducted 3 degrees, and then adducted 3 degrees. The PIP joint moved to 32 degrees of flexion; the DIP joint, 53 degrees of flexion. Initially, the fifth digit MCP joint flexed 89 degrees and abducted 17 degrees. At the end of this maneuver, the MCP joint of the fifth digit adducted 17 degrees. The PIP joint flexed 72 degrees, and the DIP joint flexed 74 degrees to complete the task.

To accomplish the first part of these motions (moving the shoulder into flexion), the shoulder joint was acted upon by concentric contractions of the anterior deltoid (primarily), trapezius, serratus anterior, coracobrachialis, and pectoralis major muscles.[1-3] These last four muscles worked as stabilizers to control the movement of the complex. Returning the shoulder complex to neutral was accomplished by eccentric contractions of the same muscles. In other words, the muscles were working in reverse to accomplish the activity in a smooth, coordinated manner.[4-5]

Flexion of the elbow joint was the result of concentric activity of the biceps brachii, brachialis, and brachioradialis muscles.[6-8] The neutral

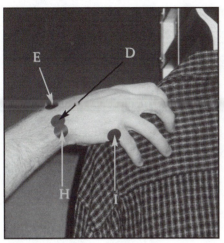

Figure 4-2. Reaching for the shirt and hanger: Close up view of the hand at the initiation of the grasp on the shirt and hanger. The key landmarks denoted by black dots are: D = ulnar head (dorsal aspect); E = radial styloid process (dorsal aspect); H = ulnar styloid process (ulnar aspect); and I = fifth MCP joint line (ulnar aspect).

position of the forearm was maintained by the synergistic activity of the supinator and pronator muscles.[9] The initial wrist motion was accomplished through concentric contractions of the extensor carpi radialii longus and brevis and extensor carpi ulnaris muscles. There was a greater contribution from the extensor carpi ulnaris muscle due to the ulnar deviation required in the early part of this motion and followed by eccentric activity to allow the flexion seen in the latter part of the motion.[10-13]

The finger activity was the result of concentric contractions of the extensors digitorum indicis, digiti minimi, and pollicis brevis and longus muscles for the extension activity and the eccentric contraction of the same muscles to accomplish the flexion activity.[14-15] Concentric contraction of the abductor pollicis longus, dorsal interossei, and abductor digiti minimi muscles allowed the abduction activity, and eccentric contraction of these same muscles allowed the adduction activity.[16] As with the shoulder complex, eccentric muscle activity was needed for controlling the motions, as the weight of the shirt was borne by the upper extremity complexes, as well as for overcoming the effects of gravity which pulled the extremity downward.[17]

DONNING THE SHIRT

With the shirt in hand, the subject proceeded to don the shirt. This portion of the activity was subdivided into two phases. The first phase included dressing the right upper extremity with the left upper extremity and then retracting the upper extremity to the side of the body to begin the second phase. The second phase included stabilization of the open shirt edge by the right upper extremity to complete the dressing of the left upper extremity.

DRESSING THE RIGHT UPPER EXTREMITY

During the first phase (Figure 4-3), the left shoulder joint moved to 38 degrees of flexion and 76 degrees of internal rotation, extended to neutral, and abducted 24 degrees.[18-20] The right shoulder joint moved to 19 degrees of flexion and 62 degrees of internal rotation. The left elbow joint moved from 77 degrees to 130 degrees of flexion and then extended to 39 degrees of flexion. The right elbow joint moved to 130 degrees of flexion. The left wrist returned to neutral, while the right wrist joint flexed 24 degrees, radially deviated 19 degrees, and then returned to 10 degrees of flexion and 4 degrees of radial deviation.

The fingers primarily flexed and abducted. Starting with the left thumb and working ulnarly, the left thumb CMC joint abducted from 18 degrees to 20 degrees and then returned to the initial 18 degrees of abduction. The thumb MCP joint extended from 33 degrees to 22 degrees of flexion and continued extending until this subphase ended at 10 degrees of flexion. The thumb IP joint started at 30 degrees of flexion and also extended by moving to 6 degrees of flexion midway through this phase and ending at 2 degrees of flexion.The remaining digits followed a similar pattern in that they decreased their amount of flexion as this subphase of the activity proceeded. The second MCP joint started at 60 degrees of flexion, decreased to 44 degrees of flexion by midphase, and ended at 19 degrees of flexion. The second PIP joint started at 70 degrees of flexion, decreased to 28 degrees of flexion, and ended at 12 degrees of flexion. The second DIP joint started at 60 degrees of flexion, decreased to 14 degrees of flexion, and ended at 7 degrees of flexion. The third MCP joint continued this pattern, starting at 74 degrees of flexion, decreasing to 60 degrees of flexion, and ending at 22 degrees of flexion. The third PIP joint started at 78 degrees of flexion, decreased to 52 degrees of flexion, and ended at 15 degrees of flexion. The third DIP joint started at 58 degrees of flexion, decreased to 10 degrees of flexion, and ended at 6 degrees of flexion.

The fourth MCP joint followed similar suit, starting at 79 degrees of flexion, decreasing to 58 degrees by midphase, and ending at 23 degrees of flexion. In addition, the MCP joint abducted 4 degrees by midphase. The fourth PIP joint moved from 2 degrees of flexion to 71 degrees of

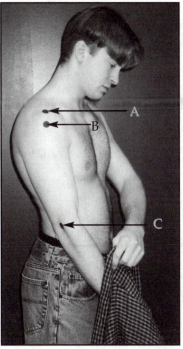

Figure 4-3. Dressing the right upper extremity: Pulling the shirt over the right hand and wrist. The key landmarks denoted by black dots are: A = acromion process (dorsal aspect); B = greater tuberosity of humerus; and C = lateral epicondyle of humerus.

flexion by midphase and ended at 24 degrees of flexion. The fourth DIP joint moved from 53 degrees of flexion to 32 degrees of flexion at midphase and continued to move to 4 degrees of flexion by endphase. The fifth MCP joint started this phase at 89 degrees of flexion, decreased to 62 degrees of flexion midway, and ended at 14 degrees of flexion. In addition, the MCP joint abducted 7 degrees by midphase. The fifth PIP joint moved from 72 to 14 degrees of flexion throughout this phase. The fifth DIP joint moved from 74 to 8 degrees of flexion throughout this phase.

Overall, the right hand followed an opposite pattern when compared to the left hand (ie, the amount of flexion increased throughout this subphase). The right thumb CMC joint started in the neutral position, moved to 6 degrees of extension at the midpoint of this subphase, and then returned to neutral. In addition, the CMC joint moved from 16 degrees of abduction to 21 degrees of abduction by midphase and then returned to the initial position of 16 degrees of abduction. The thumb MCP joint moved from 16 degrees to 12 degrees to 20 degrees of flexion throughout this phase. The thumb IP joint started at 3 degrees of flexion and maintained that position until the endphase, at which time it had reached 21 degrees of flexion.[16,21]

The second MCP joint started at 22 degrees of flexion and continued to increase throughout this phase, reaching 32 degrees and 62 degrees of flexion by mid- and endphase, respectively. The second PIP and DIP joints demonstrated similar patterns, starting at 18 degrees and moving to 32 degrees and 88 degrees of flexion and starting at 9 degrees and moving to 14 degrees and 52 degrees of flexion, respectively. The third MCP, PIP, and DIP joints also followed similar patterns by increasing their amount of flexion throughout the phase: 37 to 81 degrees of flexion for the MCP joint; 18 to 88 degrees of flexion for the PIP joint; and 2 to 44 degrees of flexion for the DIP joint. In addition, the MCP joint abducted 5 degrees by midphase and then returned to neutral by endphase.

The joints of the fourth and fifth digits increasing their flexion range of motion as the activity proceeded also followed this pattern. The fourth digit demonstrated the following ranges: MCP joint moved from 30 to 81 degrees of flexion; PIP joint moved from 24 to 72 degrees of flexion; and the DIP joint moved from 3 to 36 degrees of flexion. In addition, the fourth MCP joint reached 4 degrees of abduction by midphase and then returned to neutral by endphase. The fifth digit demonstrated the following amounts of flexion: MCP joint moved from 21 to 83 degrees; PIP joint moved from 12 to 68 degrees; and the DIP joint moved from 4 to 45 degrees of flexion. In addition, the fifth MCP joint abducted 15 degrees by midphase and returned to neutral by endphase.[22-23]

The following muscles were involved in this first phase: the subscapularis, teres major, latissimus dorsi, pectoralis major, coracobrachialis, and anterior deltoid. These muscles worked concentrically to produce the internal rotation and flexion of the left shoulder joint;[5, 24-25] the anterior deltoid and pectoralis major muscles then worked eccentrically to lower the shoulder joint; and the middle deltoid and supraspinatus muscles worked concentrically to abduct the shoulder joint. In addition, the remaining rotator cuff muscles worked eccentrically to help stabilize the glenohumeral joint.[5,26]

The anterior deltoid worked concentrically to allow the right upper extremity enough clearance from the body to don the shirt. To complete the activity, the subscapularis, teres major, latissimus dorsi, pectoralis major, coracobrachialis, and anterior deltoid muscles worked concentrically to internally rotate and flex the right shoulder.[5,24-25] The infraspinatus, teres minor, and supraspinatus muscles worked eccentrically to stabilize the movement.[5,26]

The left elbow flexors continued to work concentrically at first, then eccentrically, to complete this phase. The right elbow flexors worked concentrically to flex the elbow joint.[6-7,27]

Most of the motion during this subphase of the activity was created by the shoulder and elbow complexes. Initially, the hand continued to grasp the shirt, while the wrist joint flexed and radially deviated to bring the shirt collar over the shoulder. The muscles that provided the grasp are the same muscles that were cited in the initial phase of this overall activity. They now sustained the grasp by isometrically contracting throughout the first part of this subphase.[17,28] The left wrist muscles responsible for the flexion and radial deviation were the flexors carpi ulnaris and radialis.

Toward the end of this subphase, the grasp on the shirt collar was loosened, and the left fingers and wrist joint returned to a resting position. There was concentric contraction of the extensors digitorum communis, indicis, digiti minimi, and pollicis brevis and longus muscles of the digits, as well as concentric contractions of the fourth dorsal interossei and abductors digiti minimi and pollicis longus and brevis muscles.[17] The extensors carpi ulnaris and radialii longus and brevis muscles contracted concentrically to return the wrist joint to its neutral position.

The motion of the right hand was similar to the setting of the left hand grasp. Initially, the flexors digitorum superficialis and profundus and pollicis longus and brevis, the third and fourth dorsal interossei, and the abductors digiti minimi and pollicis longus and brevis muscles contracted concentrically to move the digits.[17] The flexor carpi radialis and ulnaris muscles contracted concentrically to move the wrist joint during the first portion of this subphase. To complete this subphase, these muscles continued to contract concentrically. In addition, the second and third palmar interossei and the second dorsal interossei muscles contracted concentrically to afford the adduction and abduction of the digits needed to fully grasp the shirt.[29]

DRESSING THE LEFT UPPER EXTREMITY

The next phase involved the left hand searching for the opening of the shirt sleeve behind the body, securing the sleeve, and bringing the left upper extremity to the front of the body to prepare for buttoning the shirt (Figures 4-4 and 4-5). To accomplish this aspect of the activity, the left shoulder joint was extended, adducted, and internally rotated, bringing the left upper extremity behind the body. The left shoulder joint started in the neutral position, hyperextended 26 degrees by midposition, and then returned to 30 degrees of flexion, bringing the shirt with it. Starting at 76 degrees of internal rotation, the left shoulder joint internally rotated another 12 degrees by midposition and then decreased to 62 degrees of internal

Figure 4-4. Dressing the left upper extremity: The left hand searching for and securing the sleeve. The key landmarks denoted by black dots are: A = acromion process (dorsal aspect); K = medial epicondyle of humerus; and L = ulnar head (ventral aspect).

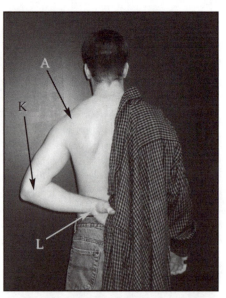

Figure 4-5. Dressing the left upper extremity: Slipping the left hand through the sleeve. The key landmarks denoted by black dots are: A = acromion process (dorsal aspect); J = olecranon process; and K = medial epicondyle of humerus.

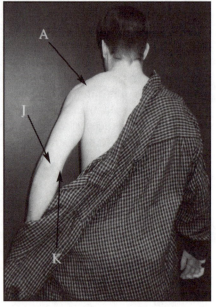

rotation at the end of this phase.[30] In addition, the left shoulder started at 24 degrees of abduction, adducted to neutral, abducted 71 degrees, and then adducted to neutral again. The right shoulder joint was in a holding position during this time, undergoing no further motion.

The left elbow joint started at 39 degrees of flexion and continued to flex to 90 degrees midway through this phase. By the end of this phase, the left elbow had returned to full extension. The right elbow joint moved from full extension to 130 degrees of flexion during this time (see Figure 4-5).

The left wrist joint flexed 61 degrees and ulnarly deviated 23 degrees by midphase. At the end of this phase, the left wrist joint was in 29 degrees of extension and had radially deviated back to neutral. The left thumb CMC joint abducted to 18 degrees; the MCP joint flexed to 10 degrees; and the IP joint flexed to 2 degrees. The left second MCP, PIP, and DIP joints flexed to 19, 12, and 7 degrees, respectively. The third MCP, PIP, and DIP joints flexed to 22, 15, and 6 degrees, respectively. The fourth MCP, PIP, and DIP joints flexed to 23, 24, and 4 degrees, respectively. The fifth MCP, PIP, and DIP joints flexed to 14, 14, and 8 degrees, respectively. All joints of the five digits maintained these positions throughout the remainder of this phase.

The right wrist joint flexed 10 degrees and radially deviated 4 degrees.[13] The right digits also flexed at all joints. The degrees of flexion seen were as follows: thumb MCP joint—20; thumb IP joint—21; second MCP joint—62; second PIP joint—88; second DIP joint—52; third MCP joint—81; third PIP joint—88; third DIP joint—44; fourth MCP joint—81; fourth PIP joint—72; fourth DIP joint—36; fifth MCP joint—82; fifth PIP joint—68; fifth DIP joint—45. In addition, the thumb CMC joint remained neutral with respect to flexion and extension and abducted 16 degrees. These positions were maintained throughout the remainder of this phase.

As the left shoulder initiated the activity of this phase of donning the shirt, the posterior deltoid, latissimus dorsi, teres major, and subscapularis muscles contracted concentrically to produce the extension, adduction, and internal rotation needed.[24-25] In addition, the subscapularis muscle helped to stabilize the shoulder joint complex during this movement. The rhomboids major and minor muscles worked concentrically to glide the scapula towards the spinous processes of the vertebral column. The pectoralis minor muscle worked concentrically to depress the point of the shoulder. The lower fibers of the trapezius muscle worked concentrically to rotate the scapula downward. The supraspinatus, infraspinatus, and teres minor muscles worked eccentrically to stabilize and control the motions occurring.[25]

To complete this phase, the arm was flexed, externally rotated, abducted, and then adducted to neutral. This was accomplished by concentric contractions of the anterior deltoid, trapezius (upper fibers), pectoralis major, infraspinatus, middle deltoid, latissimus dorsi, and teres major muscles.[31] Eccentrically, the pectoralis minor, subscapularis, and rhomboids major and minor worked to stabilize the shoulder joint complex.[26] No muscle activity was required by the right shoulder joint.

The left elbow moved from the side of the body to behind the body while increasing the amount of flexion. This motion was created by a concentric contraction of the biceps brachii, brachialis, and brachioradialis muscles. By the end of this phase, the left elbow joint, controlled by the triceps brachii and anconeus muscles acting concentrically and the biceps brachii and brachialis muscles, acting eccentrically, had returned to full extension.[32] No further muscle activity of the right elbow joint was needed at this time.

From the start of this phase to midposition, the left wrist joint and hand, searching for the shirt sleeve, traveled to the posterior portion of the body. The digits were at rest during the entire motion. The wrist joint was flexed and ulnarly deviated by concentric contractions of the flexors carpi radialis and ulnaris muscles, with the ulnaris contributing to a greater degree due to the ulnar deviation. Once in the sleeve, the wrist extended and radially deviated by concentric contractions of the extensors carpi ulnaris and radialii longus and brevis muscles, with a greater contribution from the extensors carpi radialii longus and brevis muscles due to the radial deviation.[13] Again, the digits were relaxed during this time.

Because the right hand remained grasping the shirt, the muscle activity was isometric in nature, maintained by the muscles previously cited for this component of the activity. The muscles of the forearm helped to stabilize the wrist joint and hand in this position.[17,33]

Buttoning the Shirt

The final phase of this overall activity was the buttoning of the shirt. For purposes of this activity, the buttons were secured from top to bottom, starting at the first button and working downward (Figure 4-6). The shoulder, elbow, and forearm complexes helped to precisely place the wrist and hand complexes to accomplish this task. The motions were symmetrical bilaterally. Primarily, the upper arm was stabilized as the elbow joint extended to allow the needed movements of the wrist and hand.

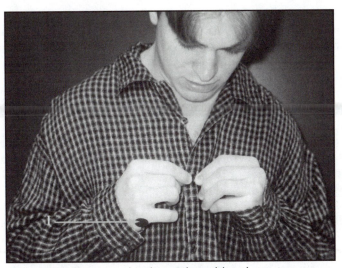

Figure 4-6. Buttoning the shirt: Bilateral hand usage to secure the first button. The key landmark denoted by the black dot is I = fifth MCP joint line (ulnar aspect).

The left shoulder joint flexed 19 degrees, internally rotated 62 degrees, and abducted 17 degrees to secure the first button. As the activity progressed downward to the other buttons, the left shoulder joint flexion decreased to 14, 10, 4, and neutral degrees, respectively. Internal rotation and abduction remained constant throughout the buttoning. The right shoulder joint demonstrated a similar pattern. The right shoulder was internally rotated 64 degrees, abducted 15 degrees, and maintained at these positions throughout this final phase. The right shoulder joint flexed to 21, 15, 10, 5 and neutral degrees, respectively, as the buttons were secured.

The left and right elbow joints started at 128 degrees of flexion and extended from start to finish, moving to 120, 109, 93, 73, and 54 degrees of flexion, respectively.

The left wrist joint started at neutral, extended to 20 degrees, and gradually increased to 29 degrees of extension by the end of the buttoning phase. There was a small amount of radial deviation throughout this phase, with the amount of deviation varying from button to button. The right wrist joint started at neutral, extended to 28 degrees, and gradually decreased to 18 degrees of extension by the end of this phase. Here too, a small amount of radial deviation occurred throughout the phase, with the amount varying from button to button.

The digits of both hands utilized a three-jaw chuck, which involves the first (thumb), second, and third digits.[14,33-35] However, this changed to a two-jaw chuck toward the end of the buttoning of each button, and then returned to a three-jaw chuck to start the next button. The fourth and fifth digits were primarily kept out of the way as the buttoning process proceeded. The main difference between left and right sides was that the left side grasped the material forming the button hole, while the right side grasped the buttons.

The majority of motion of the left digits was flexion. The thumb CMC joint abducted 14 degrees initially and decreased to 12 degrees of abduction by the end of the activity. The MCP joint flexed 12 degrees throughout the buttoning, and the IP joint remained in neutral until the end of the phase when it flexed 10 degrees. The second MCP joint flexed 58 degrees initially, decreased to 44 degrees midway, and increased to 75 degrees at the end of the phase. The PIP joint flexed to 59 degrees before fully extending at the end of the phase. The DIP joint flexed to 46 degrees before fully extending at the end of the phase as well.

The third MCP joint moved from 56 to 70 degrees of flexion. The PIP joint moved from 42 to 64 degrees of flexion before fully extending at the end. The DIP joint moved from 26 to 44 degrees of flexion before fully extending at the end. The fourth MCP flexed 12 degrees and remained the same throughout the phase. The PIP and DIP joints flexed 73 and 52 degrees, respectively, and remained the same throughout the phase. In addition, the MCP joint abducted 4 degrees and remained the same throughout the phase. The fifth MCP, PIP, and DIP joints flexed 2, 68, and 64 degrees, respectively, throughout the phase. In addition, the MCP joint abducted 16 degrees throughout the phase.

The right hand also demonstrated a predominance of flexion activity during the buttoning phase. The thumb CMC joint flexed 3 degrees and abducted 15 degrees initially. By the end of this phase, the abduction changed to 12 degrees. The MCP joint flexed to 16 degrees throughout the phase. The IP joint flexed to 30 degrees, returned to neutral by midpoint, and flexed 25 degrees at the end.

The second MCP joint flexed 64 degrees initially. It then increased to 68 degrees of flexion by midphase. By the end of the phase, flexion decreased to 62 degrees. The PIP and DIP joints moved from flexion to neutral to flexion throughout the activity. There was 28, neutral, and 28 degrees of flexion for the PIP joint; and 18, neutral, and 24 degrees of flexion for the DIP joint.

The third digit followed a similar pattern: the MCP joint flexed to 56, 70, and 66 degrees, respectively; the PIP joint flexed to 30, neutral, and 36 degrees, respectively; and the DIP joint flexed to 22, neutral, and 26 degrees, respectively.

The fourth MCP joint flexed 16 degrees and abducted 5 degrees throughout the phase. The PIP joint flexed 42 degrees and the DIP joint, 26 degrees throughout the activity. The fifth MCP joint flexed 16 degrees and abducted 18 degrees throughout the phase. The PIP joint flexed 40 degrees and the DIP joint, 26 degrees throughout the phase.

The muscles responsible for stabilizing both shoulder joint complexes were the anterior deltoid, supraspinatus, subscapularis, latissimus dorsi, teres major, pectoralis major, infraspinatus, and teres minor. The anterior deltoid and supraspinatus muscles contracted eccentrically and slowly lowered the arms as the hands traveled down the shirt. The other muscles functioned isometrically to stabilize the shoulder complexes.[5,26]

The biceps brachii, brachialis, and brachioradialis muscles worked eccentrically bilaterally to lower the forearms as the hands traveled down the shirt. These muscles momentarily switched to isometric activity as the button was maneuvered through the button hole.[6-7]

Both wrist joints were controlled by concentric contractions of the extensors carpi ulnaris and radialii longus and brevis muscles, which both extended and radially deviated the wrists. The extensors carpi radialii longus and brevis muscles contributed to a greater degree due to the radial deviation that was occurring simultaneously.[13, 36] The only change in this activity was toward the end of this phase. At that time, the right wrist joint flexed to help clear the material from the button. This was accomplished by a concentric contraction of the flexors carpi ulnaris and radialis muscles.

The left digits were controlled by the following muscles: eccentric contraction of the extensor digitorum to stabilize and control the second and third digits and to hold the fourth and fifth digits out of the way; isometric contraction of the extensor digiti minimi to hold the fifth digit out of the way; concentric, changing to isometric, contraction of the abductor digiti minimi to hold the fifth digit in position; eccentric contraction of the extensor indicis to stabilize and control the second digit; isometric contractions of the extensors and flexors pollicis longus and brevis to keep the thumb rigid; concentric contractions of the flexors digitorum superficialis and profundus to move the second through fifth digits. The opponens and adductor pollicis muscles acted concentrically to oppose and stabilize the thumb against the second and third digits. The second, third, and fourth dorsal interossei muscles and the first palmar interosseous muscle worked concentrically as the digits grasped the material.[17,29,37-38]

As the activity progressed to the endphase, first and second lumbricals contracted concentrically to flex the MCP joint and extend the PIP and DIP joints of the respective digits.[29] The second dorsal interosseous and first palmar interosseous muscles worked concentrically to keep the second and third digits approximated to each other. The activity of the opponens pollicis muscle changed to isometric contraction to maintain the grasp with the second digit. The flexor pollicis longus changed to concentric contraction to help push the button through the button hole.

At the beginning of this phase, the muscle activity of the right hand was similar to that of the left hand. By midphase, the right extensors pollicis longus and digitorum muscles worked concentrically to extend the IP joint of the thumb and the PIP and DIP joints of the second and third digits.

Toward the endphase, the first and second lumbricals contracted concentrically to flex the MCP joint and extend the PIP and DIP joints of the respective digits. The second dorsal interosseous and the first palmar interosseous muscles worked concentrically to keep the second and third digits approximated. The adductor pollicis and the flexor pollicis longus muscles acted concentrically to stabilize the digit and to flex the IP joint of the thumb. The opponens pollicis muscle worked isometrically to maintain the grasp.[16]

SUMMARY

Key Anatomical Landmarks for Shirt Analysis

Shoulder Complex:	Greater tuberosity of humerus
	Acromion process (dorsal aspect)
Elbow and Forearm Complex:	Lateral epicondyle of humerus
	Medial epicondyle of humerus
	Olecranon process
	Radial styloid process (dorsal aspect)
	Radial styloid process (radial aspect)
	Ulnar head (dorsal aspect)
	Ulnar styloid process (ulnar aspect)
Wrist and Hand Complex:	Base of first MCP (radial and palmar aspects)
	Base of second MCP (dorsal aspect)
	Base of fifth MCP (dorsal aspect)
	First MCP joint line (palmar aspect)
	Second MCP joint line (radial aspect)
	Fifth MCP joint line (ulnar aspect)
	First IP joint line (palmar aspect)
	Second PIP joint line (radial aspect)

Fifth PIP joint line (ulnar aspect)
Second DIP joint line (radial aspect)
Fifth DIP joint line (ulnar aspect)

Major Phases for Shirt Analysis

Starting Position

- Position of subject

- Height of hanger

- Distance of subject from hanger

- Type of shirt

Removing the Shirt from a Hanger

Donning the Shirt

- Dressing the right upper extremity

- Dressing the left upper extremity

Buttoning the Shirt

Upper Extremity Motions and Muscular Activity: Donning and Buttoning a Shirt

Introduction and Set-Up

- All joints are in the anatomical position at the start of the activity with the exception of the radioulnar joints which are midway between supination and pronation.

Removing the Shirt From a Hanger

- Primarily flexion of all joints.

- Extension of the second and third MCP joints.

- Abduction of the thumb CMC joint.

- Primarily concentric contractions of proximal muscles.

- Eccentric contractions of distal muscles.

Dressing the Right Upper Extremity

• Primarily flexion and internal rotation of the shoulder joints.

• Flexion of the elbow joints and right wrist joint.

• Extension of the left wrist joint and left digits.

• Flexion of the right digits.

• Primarily concentric contractions of all muscles.

Dressing the Left Upper Extremity

• Primarily extension of left shoulder with flexion of the distal joints.

• All concentric muscular contractions.

• Right shoulder and elbow are maintaining their positions via isometric muscular activity.

Buttoning the Shirt

• Primarily flexion and internal rotation of the shoulder joints.

• Flexion of the elbow joints and extension of the wrist joints.

• Flexion of the distal joints.

• Primarily concentric muscular contractions.

• Primarily isometric muscular contractions for PIP and DIP joints of digits four and five.

CLINICAL APPLICATION AND STUDY QUESTIONS

This analysis demonstrated one way of donning and buttoning a shirt. Obviously, the biomechanics would change with different types of shirts. Discuss the changes that would be noted with a female-tailored shirt, a male- or female-zippered shirt, and a pullover top. How does the donning of a shirt differ if most of the buttons are secured first and then the shirt is pulled over the head and torso? What effect would different types of materials have on this activity?

Make a list of possible muscle substitutions for the primary muscles involved in this activity. Compare your list to Chart 1 in Appendix A.

Discuss any assistive devices that would be of value in buttoning a shirt.

According to Perry, through the many combinations of movement available at the shoulder, elbow, and forearm complexes, there are approximately 2 million different possibilities for hand placement.[1] Individuals tend to vary their ADL performances on a daily basis, which may help prevent repetitive motion-type injuries and/or lessen the extent of such injuries. What other ways of donning a shirt can you demonstrate?

REFERENCES

1. Perry T. Normal upper extremity kinesiology. *Phys Ther.* 1978;58:165-178.

2. Culham E, Peat M. Functional anatomy of the shoulder complex. *J Orthop Sports Phys Ther.* 1993;18:342-350.

3. Dvir Z, Berme N. The shoulder complex in elevation of the arm: a mechanism approach. *J Biomech.* 1978;11:219-225.

4. Kent BE. Functional anatomy of the shoulder complex: a review. *Phys Ther.* 1971;51:867-888.

5. Kronberg M, Nemeth G, Brostrom L. Muscle activity and coordination in the normal shoulder. *Clin Orthop.* 1990;257:76-85.

6. An KN, Hui FC, Morrey BF, Linscheid RL, Chao EY. Muscles across the elbow joint: a biomechanical analysis. *J Biomech.* 1981;14:659-669.

7. Basmajian JV, Letif A. Integrated actions and functions of the chief flexors of the elbow: a detailed electromyographic analysis. *J Bone Joint Surg Am.* 1957;39:1106-1118.

8. Morrey BF, Askew LJ, An KN, Chao EY. A biomechanical study of normal and functional elbow motion. *J Bone Joint Surg Am.* 1981;63:872-877.

9. Ray RD, Johnson RJ, Jameson RM. Rotation of the forearm: an experimental study of pronation and supination. *J Bone Joint Surg Am.* 1951;33:993-996.

10. Brumfield RH, Champoux JA. A biomechanical study of normal functional wrist motion. *Clin Orthop.* 1979;187:23-25.

11. Backdahl M, Carlsöö S. Distribution of activity in muscles acting on the wrist. *Acta Morphologica Neerlando-Scandinavica.* 1961;4:136-141.

12. Sarrafian SK, Melamed JL, Goshgarian GM. Study of wrist motion in flexion and extension. *Clin Orthop.* 1977;126:153-159.

13. Youm Y, McMurty RY, Flatt AE, Gillespie TE. Kinematics of the wrist. I. An experimental study of radial-ulnar deviation and flexion-extension. *J Bone Joint Surg Am.* 1978;60:423-432.

14. An KN, Chao EY, Cooney WP, Linscheid RI. Normative model of human hand for biomechanical analysis. *J Biomech*. 1979;12:775-788.

15. Brand PW, Cranor KC, Ellis JC. Tendon and pulleys at the metacarpophalangeal joint of a finger. *J Bone Joint Surg Am*. 1975;57:779-784.

16. Iameda T, An K, Cooney WP. Functional anatomy and biomechanics of the thumb. *Hand Clin*. 1992;8:9-15.

17. Long C, Conrad PW, Hall EA, Furler SL. Intrinsic-extrinsic muscle control of the hand in power grip and precision handling: an electromyographic study. *J Bone Joint Surg Br*. 1970;52:853-867.

18. Blakely RL, Palmer ML. Analysis of rotation accompanying shoulder flexion. *Phys Ther*. 1984;64:1214-1216.

19. Browne AO, An KN, Tanaka S, Morrey BF. Glenohumeral elevation studied in three dimensions. *J Bone Joint Surg Br*. 1990;72:843-845.

20. Quiring DP, Boroush EL. Functional anatomy of the shoulder girdle. *Arch Phys Med Rehabil*. 1946;27:90-96.

21. Barmakian JT. Anatomy of the joints of the thumb. *Hand Clin*. 1992;683-691.

22. Craig SM. Anatomy of the joints of the fingers. *Hand Clin*. 1992;8:693-700.

23. Youm Y, Gillespie TE, Flatt AE, Sprague BL. Kinematic investigation of normal MCP joint. *J Biomech*. 1978;11:109-118.

24. Broome HL, Basmajian JV. The function of the teres major muscle: an electromyographic study. *Anat Rec*. 1970;170:309-310.

25. Nemeth G, Kronberg M, Brostrom L. Electromyogram (EMG) recordings from the subscapularis muscle: description of a technique. *J Orthop Res*. 1990;8:151-153.

26. Saha AK. Dynamic stability of the glenohumeral joint. *Acta Orthop Scand*. 1971;42:491-505.

27. Ober AG. An electromyographic analysis of elbow flexors during submaximal concentric contractions. *Res Q Exerc Sport*. 1988;59:139-143.

28. Chao EY, Opgrande JD, Axmear FE. Three-dimensional force analysis of finger joints in selected isometric hand functions. *J Biomech*. 1976;9:387-396.

29. Sunderland S. Actions of the extensor digitorum communis, interosseous, and lumbrical muscles. *Am J Anat*. 1945;77:189-194.

30. Howell SM, Galinat BJ, Renzi AJ. Normal and abnormal biomechanics of the glenohumeral joint in the horizontal plane. *J Bone Joint Surg Am*. 1988;70:227-232.

31. Walmsley RP, Szybbo C. A comparative study of the torque generated by the shoulder internal and external rotator muscles in different positions and at varying speeds. *J Orthop Sports Phys Ther*. 1987;9:217-222.

32. Basmajian JV, Griffin WR. Function of anconeus muscle: an electromyographic study. *J Bone Joint Surg Am*. 1972;54:1712-1714.

33. Jones LA. The assessment of hand function: a critical review of techniques. *J Hand Surg Am*. 1989;14:221-228.

34. Buchholz B, Armstrong TJ. A kinematic model of the human hand to evaluate its prehensile abilities. *J Biomech.* 1992;25:149-162.

35. Landsmeer JMF. Power grip and precision handling. *Ann Rheum Dis.* 1962;21:164-170.

36. Radonjic D, Long CL. Kinesiology of the wrist. *Am J Phys Med Rehabil.* 1971;50:57-71.

37. An KN, Chao EY, Cooney WP, Linscheid RI. Tendon excursion and moment arm of index finger muscles. *J Biomech.* 1983;16:419-426.

38. Long C, Brown ME. Electromyographic kinesiology of the hand: muscles moving the long finger. *J Bone Joint Surg Am.* 1964;46:1683-1686.

SUGGESTED READINGS

An KN, Browne AO, Tanaka S, Morrey BF. Three-dimensional kinematics of glenohumeral elevation. *J Orthop Res.* 1991;9:143-149.

Basset RW, Browne AO, Morrey BF, An KN. Glenohumeral muscle force and moment mechanics in a position of shoulder instability. *J Biomech.* 1990;23:405-412.

Gerdle B, Elert J, Henriksson-Larsen K. Muscular fatigue during repeated isokinetic shoulder forward flexions in young females. *Eur J Appl Physiol.* 1988;57:415-419.

Hagberg M. Workload and fatigue in repetitive arm elevations. *Ergonomics.* 1981;24:543-555.

Hagberg M. Electromyographic signs of shoulder muscular fatigue in two elevated arm positions. *Am J Phys Med Rehabil.* 1981;60:111-121.

Herberts P, Kadefors R, Broman H. Arm positioning in manual tasks—an electromyographic study of localized muscle fatigue. *Ergonomics.* 1980;23:655-665.

Kauer JMG. Functional anatomy of the wrist. *Clin Orthop.* 1980;149:9-20.

Provins KA, Salter N. Maximum torque exerted about the elbow joint. *J Appl Physiol.* 1955;7:393-398.

Ryu J, Cooney WP, Askew LJ, An KN, Chao EYS. Functional ranges of motion of the wrist joint. *J Hand Surg Am.* 1991;16:409-419.

Shiffman LM. Effects of aging on adult hand function. *Am J Occup Ther.* 1992;46:785-791.

Stroyan M, Wilk KE. The functional anatomy of the elbow complex. *J Orthop Sports Phys Ther.* 1993;17:279-288.

Tarbert JA, Wolin PM. Rotator cuff. *Phys and Sports Med J.* 1997;25:54-74.

Wadsworth CT. Clinical anatomy and mechanics of the wrist and hand. *J Orthop Sports Phys Ther.* 1983;4:206-216.

Chapter 5

Sweeping With a Broom

INTRODUCTION AND SET-UP

There are many types of brooms for sweeping surfaces. A few examples are a push broom with a wooden handle, a standard broom with a wooden handle, a set with a short broom, a long-handled dustpan (intended to prevent bending over to pick up debris), and a whisk-type broom with a short wooden handle. This analysis looked at the motions of the upper extremity in using a standard broom with a wooden handle. The wooden handle was 52½ inches long with a diameter of 2¾ inches and was attached to a set of bristles that spanned 12½ inches across the bottom (the portion that interfaces with the surface being swept). The activity was divided into five phases: 1) reaching for the broom; 2) grasping the broom; 3) bringing the broom into position for sweeping; 4) reaching to sweep; and 5) sweeping.

REACHING FOR THE BROOM

The subject was standing in the anatomical position facing the broom as the analysis began. The subject reached forward with the right upper extremity to get the broom (Figure 5-1). The scapula abducted and rotated upward as the glenohumeral joint forward flexed 25 degrees. The elbow joint flexed 10 degrees and the forearm pronated 45 degrees.

The scapular motion was achieved through a concentric contraction of the serratus anterior muscle. The anterior deltoid and the coracobrachialis muscles worked concentrically to achieve the forward flexion of the shoulder joint.[1-3] The elbow joint motion was brought about by a concentric contraction of the brachialis muscle.[4-5] The pronators teres and quadratus muscles worked concentrically to bring the forearm into its pronated position.[6]

Figure 5-1. Reaching for the broom: Subject has grasped the broom. The key landmarks denoted by black dots are: A = acromion process; B = greater tuberosity of humerus; C = lateral epicondyle of humerus; D = ulnar head (dorsal aspect); E = radial styloid process (dorsal aspect); and H = ulnar styloid process (ulnar aspect).

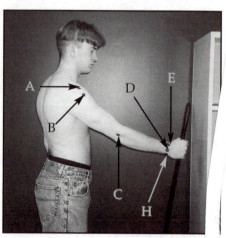

GRASPING THE BROOM

The right wrist and hand complexes were brought into play as t subject grasped the broom (Figure 5-2). The right wrist joint was radi: ly deviated 5 to 10 degrees while being maintained in a position mi way between flexion and extension.[7]

The first CMC joint flexed 85 degrees and abducted 40 degrees, whi the MCP joint flexed 75 degrees, and the IP joint flexed 55 degrees. On positioned around the broom handle, the thumb adducted 5 degrees i oppose the broom handle. The second MCP joint flexed 80 degrees; th PIP joint, 90 degrees; and the DIP joint, 60 degrees. The third MCP join flexed 95 degrees; the PIP joint, 100 degrees; and the DIP joint, 6 degrees. The fourth MCP joint flexed 100 degrees; the PIP joint, 9 degrees; and the DIP joint, 75 degrees. The fifth MCP joint flexed 10(degrees; the PIP joint, 85 degrees; and the DIP joint, 50 degrees.[8-9]

The flexor carpi radialis and the extensors carpi radialii longus and brevis muscles worked concentrically to bring the wrist into position to grasp the broom.[10] The muscular activity of the digits was concentric in nature and worked as follows: the flexors pollicis longus and brevis and the abductors pollicis longus and brevis muscles positioned the first digit; this was followed by contraction of the adductor pollicis muscle. The flexors digitorum superficialis and profundus, along with the lumbricals and the interossei muscles, controlled the flexion component of the second through fifth digits.[11-12]

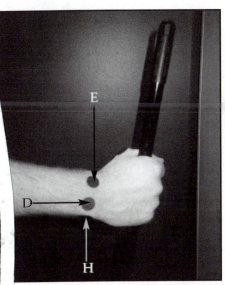

Figure 5-2. Grasp of the broom: Close-up view of cylindrical power grip. The key landmarks denoted by black dots are: D = ulnar head (dorsal aspect); E = radial styloid process (dorsal aspect); and H = ulnar styloid process (ulnar aspect).

BRINGING THE BROOM INTO POSITION FOR SWEEPING

Once the broom had been grasped, the subject positioned the broom for sweeping. This phase was divided into two subphases: subphase A was the drawing of the broom in toward the body, and subphase B was grasping the broom handle by the opposite extremity.

Subphase A: Drawing the Broom in Toward the Body—Right Upper Extremity

Subphase A, drawing the broom in toward the body by the right upper extremity (Figure 5-3), began with the scapula adducting, while the glenohumeral joint extended 25 degrees from the flexed posture of phase 1. (This brought the arm back to its starting position.) In addition, the glenohumeral joint internally rotated 29 degrees. The elbow joint continued to flex another 79 degrees to come to 89 degrees of flexion by the end of this phase. The forearm remained in the same posture as in phase 1. The digits maintained their grasp on the broom handle.

The rhomboids major and minor worked concentrically to adduct the scapula. The posterior deltoid and latissimus dorsi muscles worked concentrically to extend the glenohumeral joint. The internal rotation was achieved through concentric activity of the latissimus dorsi, teres major, and subscapularis muscles.[13-16] The additional flexion of the elbow joint was brought about by a concentric contraction of the brachialis muscle.

Figure 5-3. Drawing the broom toward the body: The right upper extremity grasped the broom and moved it closer to the front of the body. The key landmarks denoted by black dots are: A = acromion process; B = greater tuberosity of humerus; C = lateral epicondyle of humerus; D = ulnar head (dorsal aspect); E = radial styloid process (dorsal aspect); and H = ulnar styloid process (ulnar aspect).

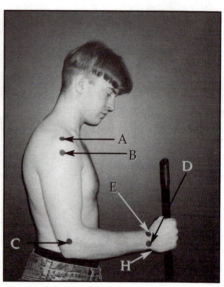

The forearm and hand muscles functioned isometrically to maintain the wrist joint and digit posture of the previous phase.

Subphase B: Grasping of the Broom Handle— Opposite Extremity

The opposite extremity (the left in this analysis) reached for the broom handle in order to commence sweeping (Figure 5-4). Starting in the anatomical position, the left shoulder joint was flexed 25 degrees and internally rotated 29 degrees, similar to the activity of the right-sided joints seen in the previous phase.

The elbow joint flexed 10 degrees, and the forearm pronated 45 degrees. The wrist joint radially deviated 17 degrees while being maintained in a neutral position midway between flexion and extension. The digits of the hand followed a similar pattern to the activity of the right-sided digits, which were described previously.

The muscular activity for this entire subphase was similar to the activity of the right upper extremity. The main difference was the flexion and internal rotation components of the left shoulder joint. This motion was brought about by concentric contractions of the pectoralis major and subscapularis muscles.[15] As the pectoralis major is capable of drawing the shoulder joint into a forward flexion component, there was less need for the anterior deltoid and coracobrachialis muscles in the left upper extremity.

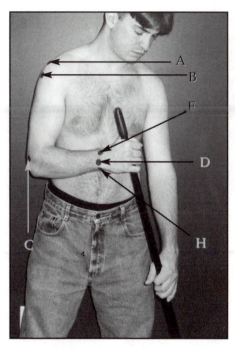

Figure 5-4. Grasping the broom with the opposite extremity: Left hand positioned to begin sweeping. The key landmarks denoted by black dots are: A = acromion process; B = greater tuberosity of humerus; C = lateral epicondyle of humerus; D = ulnar head (dorsal aspect); E = radial styloid process (dorsal aspect); and H = ulnar styloid process (ulnar aspect).

REACHING TO SWEEP

As with the previous phase, this phase of reaching to sweep was divided into subphase A and subphase B. Subphase A was reaching with the left upper extremity in preparation for the actual sweeping motion. Subphase B was sweeping from the left side to the right side.

Subphase A: Reaching with the Left Upper Extremity

The left shoulder joint was abducted 5 degrees (Figure 5-5). The elbow joint was maintained in the position assumed when the broom was grasped. The wrist joint remained in its radially deviated position of the last phase. The digits maintained their grasp on the broom handle.

The middle deltoid and supraspinatus muscles acted concentrically to abduct the shoulder joint.[17] The triceps brachii, anconeus, and biceps brachii muscles worked synergistically to maintain the position of the elbow.[18-19] The extensors carpi radialis and carpi radialii longus and brevis muscles worked synergistically to maintain the wrist position. The muscular activity of the digits remained the same as in the last phase.

Figure 5-5. Sweeping from left to right: The left shoulder joint horizontally adducted while the left elbow joint flexed. The key landmarks denoted by black dots are: A = acromion process; B = greater tuberosity of humerus; D = ulnar head (dorsal aspect); E = radial styloid process (dorsal aspect); H = ulnar styloid process (ulnar aspect); and I = fifth MCP joint line (ulnar aspect).

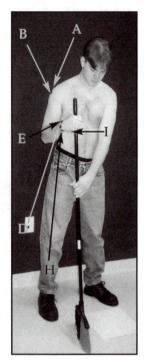

Subphase B: Sweeping from the Left Side to the Right Side

The left shoulder joint horizontally adducted 20 to 25 degrees, abducting the scapula 17 degrees[20] (Figure 5-6). The elbow joint flexed 25 degrees to bring the elbow joint into 35 degrees of flexion by the end of this subphase. The forearm supinated approximately 5 degrees. The wrist joint radially deviated another 5 degrees. The digits maintained their grasp on the broom handle.

The pectoralis major and minor muscles worked concentrically to horizontally adduct the shoulder joint. The biceps brachii and the brachialis muscles worked concentrically to flex the elbow. The biceps brachii muscle worked concentrically to supinate the wrist joint. The flexor carpi radialis and the extensors carpi radialii longus and brevis worked concentrically to achieve the additional radial deviation of the wrist joint. The muscles of the digits continued to work isometrically to maintain the grasp on the broom handle.[12,21]

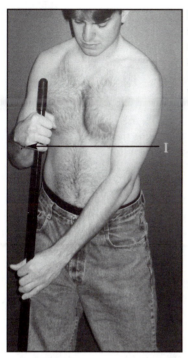

Figure 5-6. Sweep of the right arm: The shoulder joint adducted and internally rotated while the elbow joint was flexed and the wrist ulnarly deviated. The key landmark denoted by the black dot is I = fifth MCP joint line (ulnar aspect).

SWEEPING

The sweeping phase of this activity was a repetitive motion, proceeding from the subject's left side toward the right side, and then back again to prepare for the next sweeping motion. As in the previous two phases, the sweeping phase was divided into subphase A: the sweep of the left arm, and subphase B: the sweep of the right arm.

Subphase A: The Sweep of the Left Arm

The left shoulder horizontally abducted 110 degrees, while the scapula adducted and rotated downward. The elbow joint flexed to 95 degrees. The forearm pronated 45 degrees. The wrist joint ulnarly deviated to neutral. The digits maintained their grasp on the broom handle.

The posterior deltoid muscle worked concentrically to horizontally abduct the shoulder joint. The brachialis, biceps brachii, and brachioradialis muscles worked concentrically to flex the elbow joint. The pronators teres and quadratus muscles pronated the forearm through concentric activity. The flexor carpi radialis and the extensors carpi radialii longus and brevis worked eccentrically to return the wrist joint to neutral from its previously radially deviated position. The muscles of the digits continued to work isometrically to maintain the grasp on the broom.

Subphase B: The Sweep of the Right Arm

The right shoulder joint was adducted 60 degrees, while the scapula adducted and rotated downward. In addition, the shoulder joint was internally rotated 30 degrees. The elbow joint was flexed to 120 degrees. The wrist ulnarly deviated 20 degrees. The digits maintained their grasp (see Figure 5-6).

The pectoralis major and minor, the latissimus dorsi, and the teres major muscles worked concentrically to produce the motion at the shoulder joint. The brachialis, biceps brachii, and brachioradialis muscles worked concentrically to flex the elbow joint. Eccentric contractions of the flexor carpi radialis and the extensors carpi radialii longus and brevis muscles ulnarly deviated the wrist.[10] The muscular activity of the digits continued isometrically.

To continue sweeping and complete the task, the subject alternated between the last two phases. In some instances, the subject may switch posture and sweep from right to left across the surface being swept. In this case, the motions and muscular activity would be reversed. The activity noted for the left upper extremity would become that of the right upper extremity and vice versa.

SUMMARY

Key Anatomical Landmarks for Sweeping Analysis

Shoulder Complex:	Greater tuberosity of humerus
	Acromion process (dorsal aspect)
Elbow and Forearm Complex:	Lateral epicondyle of humerus
	Radial styloid process (dorsal aspect)
	Radial styloid process (radial aspect)
	Ulnar head (dorsal aspect)
	Ulnar styloid process (ulnar aspect)
Wrist and Hand Complex:	Base of first MCP (radial and palmar aspects)
	Base of second MCP (dorsal aspect)
	Base of fifth MCP (dorsal aspect)
	First MCP joint line (palmar aspect)

Second MCP joint line (radial aspect)
Fifth MCP joint line (ulnar aspect)
First IP joint line (palmar aspect)
Second PIP joint line (radial aspect)
Fifth PIP joint line (ulnar aspect)
Second DIP joint line (radial aspect)
Fifth DIP joint line (ulnar aspect)

Major Phases for Sweeping Analysis

Starting Position

• Position of subject

• Type of broom

Reaching for the Broom

Grasping the Broom

Bringing the Broom into Position for Sweeping

• Drawing the broom in toward the body—right upper
extremity

• Grasping of the broom handle—opposite extremity

Reaching to Sweep

• Reaching with the left upper extremity

• Sweeping from the left side to the right side

Sweeping

• The sweep of the left arm

• The sweep of the right arm

Upper Extremity Joint Motions and Muscular Activity: Sweeping With a Broom

Introduction and Set-Up

• Subject is standing in the anatomical position, facing the
broom.

Reaching for the Broom

- Flexion of the shoulder and elbow joint.

- Pronation of the radioulnar joint.

- All concentric muscular activity.

Grasping the Broom

- Radial deviation of the wrist joint.

- Flexion of the digits.

- All concentric muscular activity.

Bringing the Broom into Position for Sweeping

Drawing the broom in toward the body—right upper extremity

- Extension and internal rotation of the shoulder joint.

- Flexion of the elbow joint.

- All concentric activity for shoulder and elbow muscles.

- All other joints are maintaining their positions via isometric muscular activity.

Bringing the Broom into Position for Sweeping

Grasping of the broom handle—opposite extremity

- Flexion of shoulder and elbow joints.

- Pronation of radioulnar joint

- Radial deviation of wrist joint.

- All concentric muscular activity.

- Digits are maintaining their positions via isometric muscular contraction.

Reaching to Sweep—Reach With the Left Upper Extremity

- Abduction of shoulder via concentric muscle activity.

- All other joints are maintaining their positions via isometric muscular activity.

Reaching to Sweep—Sweeping from the Left Side to the Right Side

- Horizontal adduction of shoulder joint.

- Elbow flexion, radioulnar supination, and wrist radial deviation.

- All concentric activity of muscles.

- Digits are maintaining their positions via isometric muscular activity.

Sweeping—The Sweep of the Left Arm

- Horizontal abduction of shoulder.

- Elbow flexion, radioulnar pronation, and wrist ulnar deviation.

- Primarily concentric muscular contractions.

- Digits are maintaining their positions via isometric muscular activity.

Sweeping—The Sweep of the Right Arm

- Adduction and internal rotation of the shoulder joint.

- Elbow flexion and wrist ulnar deviation.

- Primarily concentric muscular activity.

- Digits are maintaining their positions via isometric muscular activity.

CLINICAL APPLICATION AND DISCUSSION QUESTIONS

This activity was based on the use of a standard wooden-handled broom. The activity would change if the other types of brooms cited at the beginning of this chapter were used. The other variation in this activity would be the type of surface being swept, with a more erosive surface requiring more muscular activity.

Discuss the muscle activity if a push broom was used. How do the upper extremity motions differ? What happens muscularly if a whisk-type broom is used?

How would this compare with using a rake to gather leaves or other fallen debris? Is the hand grip the same? Are the motions the same? Is the force needed to control the rake the same? Does the type of rake used make a difference in the muscular activity? How does the use of a garden hoe change the activity analysis? What other activities utilize comparable upper extremity motions and muscular activities?

Make a list of injuries and/or medical conditions that would interfere with the normal performance of this activity. List muscle substitutions for the primary muscles in this analysis and compare the list to Chart 1 in Appendix A.

REFERENCES

1.   Browne AO, An KN, Tanaka S, Morrey BF. Glenohumeral elevation studied in three dimensions. *J Bone Joint Surg Br*. 1990;72:843-845.
2.   Culham E, Peat M. Functional anatomy of the shoulder complex. *J Orthop Sports Phys Ther*. 1993;18:342-350.
3.   Dvir Z, Berme N. The shoulder complex in elevation of the arm: a mechanism approach. *J Biomech*. 1978;11:219-225.
4.   Basmajian JV, Latif A. Integrated actions and functions of the chief flexors of the elbow: a detailed electromyographic analysis. *J Bone Joint Surg Am*. 1957;39:1106-1118.
5.   Ober AG. An electromyographic analysis of elbow flexors during submaximal concentric contractions. *Res Q Exerc Sport*. 1988;59:139-143.
6.   Ray RD, Johnson RJ, Jameson RM. Rotation of the forearm: an experimental study of pronation and supination. *J Bone Joint Surg Am*. 1951;33:993-996.
7.   Brumfield RH, Champoux JA. A biomechanical study of normal functional wrist motion. *Clin Orthop*. 1979;187:23-25.
8.   An KN, Chao EY, Cooney WP, Linscheid RI. Normative model of human hand for biomechanical analysis. *J Biomech*. 1979;12:775-788.

9. Buchholz B, Armstrong TJ. A kinematic model of the human hand to evaluate its prehensile abilities. *J Biomech.* 1992;25:149-162.

10. Youm Y, McMurty RY, Flatt AE, Gillespie TE. Kinematics of the wrist. I. An experimental study of radial-ulnar deviation and flexion-extension. *J Bone Joint Surg Am.* 1978;60:423-432.

11. Jones LA. The assessment of hand function: a critical review of techniques. *J Hand Surg Am.* 1989;14:221-228.

12. Long C, Conrad PW, Hall EA, Furler SL. Intrinsic-extrinsic muscle control of   the hand in power grip and precision handling: an electromyographic study. *J Bone Joint Surg Br.* 1970;52:853-867.

13. Broome HL, Basmajian JV. The function of the teres major muscle: an electromyographic study. *Anat Rec.* 1970;170:309-310.

14. Kronberg M, Nemeth G, Brostrom L. Muscle activity and coordination in the normal shoulder. *Clin Orthop.* 1990;257:76-85.

15. Nemeth G, Kronberg M, Brostrom L. Electromyogram (EMG) recordings from the subscapularis muscle: description of a technique. *J Orthop Res.* 1990;8:151-153.

16. Walmsley RP, Szybbo C. A comparative study of the torque generated by the shoulder internal and external rotator muscles in different positions and at varying speeds. *J Orthop Sports Phys Ther.* 1987;9:217-222.

17. Howell SM, Imoberseg AM, Seger DH, Marone PJ. Clarification of the role of the supraspinatus muscle in shoulder function. *J Bone Joint Surg Am.* 1985;68:398-404.

18. An KN, Hui FC, Morrey BF, Linscheid RL, Chao EY. Muscles across the elbow joint: a biomechanical analysis. *J Biomech.* 1981;14:659-669.

19. Basmajian JV, Griffin WR. Function of anconeus muscle: an electromyographic study. *J Bone Joint Surg Am.* 1972;54:1712-1714.

20. Howell SM, Galinat BJ, Renzi AJ. Normal and abnormal mechanics of the glenohumeral joint in the horizontal plane. *J Bone Joint Surg Am.* 1988;70:227-232.

21. Chao EY, Opgrande JD, Axmear FE. Three-dimensional force analysis of finger joints in selected isometric hand functions. *J Biomech.* 1976;9:387-396.

SUGGESTED READINGS

Atkeson CG. Learning arm kinematics and dynamics. *Annu Rev Neurosci.* 1989;12:157-183.

Ayoub MM, LoPresti P. The determination of an optimum size cylindrical handle by use of electromyography. *Ergonomics.* 1971;4:503-518.

Bechtol C. Biomechanics of the shoulder. *Clin Orthop.* 1980;146:37-41.

Engen TJ, Spencer WA. Method of kinematic study of normal upper extremity movements. *Arch Phys Med Rehabil.* 1968;49:9-11.

Gerdle B, Elert J, Henriksson-Larsen K. Muscular fatigue during repeated isokinetic shoulder forward flexions in young females. *Eur J Appl Physiol.* 1988;57:415-419.

Hagberg M. Electromyographic signs of shoulder muscular fatigue in two elevated arm positions. *Am J Phys Med Rehabil.* 1981;60:111-121.

Hagberg M. Workload and fatigue in repetitive arm elevations. *Ergonomics.* 1981;24:543-555.

Herberts P, Kadefors R, Broman H. Arm positioning in manual tasks— electromyographic study of localized muscle fatigue. *Ergonomics.* 1980;23:655-665.

Hsia PT, Drury CG. A simple method of evaluating handle design. *Appl Ergonomics.* 1986;17:209-213.

Ishizuki M. Functional anatomy of the elbow joint and three-dimensional quantitative analysis of the elbow joint. *Journal of the Japanese Orthopedic Association.* 1979;53:986-989.

Kauer JMG. Functional anatomy of the wrist. *Clin Orthop.* 1980;149:9-20.

Landsmeer JMF. Power grip and precision handling. *Ann Rheum Dis.* 1962;21:164-170.

Morrey BF, Askew LJ, An KN, Chao EY. A biomechanical study of normal and functional elbow motion. *J Bone Joint Surg Am.* 1981;63:872-877.

Peat M. Functional anatomy of the shoulder complex. *Phys Ther.* 1986;66:1855-1865.

Perry T. Normal upper extremity kinesiology. *Phys Ther.* 1978;58:165-178.

Saha AK. Dynamic stability of the glenohumeral joint. *Acta Orthop Scand.* 1971;42:491-505.

Stern EB. Wrist extensor orthoses: dexterity and grip strength across four styles. *Am J Occup Ther.* 1991;45:42-48.

Stroyan M, Wilk KE. The functional anatomy of the elbow complex. *J Orthop Sports Phys Ther.* 1993;17:279-288.

Taylor CL, Schwarz RJ. The anatomy and mechanics of the human hand. *Artificial Limbs.* 1955;2:22-34.

Volz RG, Lieb M, Benjamin J. Biomechanics of the wrist. *Clin Orthop.* 1980;149:112-117.

Wadsworth CT. Clinical anatomy and mechanics of the wrist and hand. *J Orthop Sports Phys Ther.* 1983;4:206-216.

Chapter 6

Donning an Ankle-Length Sock

Introduction and Set-Up

There are many ways in which people don their socks. Some people sit and bring the upper extremity to the foot; others sit and bring the foot toward the upper extremity; and others stand and prop the foot being dressed on a bed or chair and bring the upper extremity toward the foot. In any of these situations, the activity of the upper extremity becomes a key component of the task. The amount of motion needed varies with the length of the sock being donned, as well as the texture and weave of the material from which the sock is made.

For the purpose of this analysis, the subject was seated in a straight back chair with the hip and knee joints in 90 degrees of flexion, the ankle joint in neutral, and the feet resting on the floor. Both upper extremities were resting on the lap, with the shoulder joints flexed 5 degrees and internally rotated 45 degrees, the elbow joints flexed to 75 degrees, the forearms pronated 10 degrees, the left wrist in neutral, the right wrist flexed 5 degrees, and the fingers in a resting position (minimum flexion of all digits). The sock being donned was ankle-length and held in the left hand. The sock was draped over the second digit, lying between the thumb and the second digit (Figure 6-1).

The subject bent over and placed the sock on the right foot, with the majority of the motion being derived from the upper extremities. Upon donning the sock, the subject returned to the upright seated position. For a better understanding of the intricacies of this activity, the analysis was divided into four phases: 1) grasping the sock, 2) bringing the sock to the toes of the foot, 3) placing the sock over the heel of the foot and lower leg, and 4) return of the subject to the starting position.

Figure 6-1. Starting position: Subject seated, holding sock in left hand. The key landmarks denoted by black dots are: A = acromion process; B = greater tuberosity of humerus; D = ulnar head (dorsal aspect); E = radial styloid process (dorsal aspect); and F = radial styloid process (radial aspect).

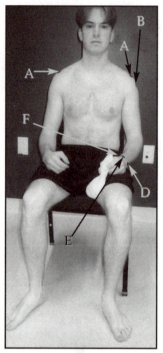

GRASPING THE SOCK

The first phase covered the motion of the upper extremities from the starting position to grasping the sock with the right and left hands (Figure 6-2). There was simultaneous horizontal adduction (too minimal to be measured) of both shoulder joints to bring the hands toward each other.[1] The elbows maintained their initial position. The left forearm pronated 5 degrees, while the right forearm remained in neutral. The left wrist extended 15 degrees, and the right wrist extended 5 degrees. Initially, the left thumb abducted 10 degrees and then adducted 15 degrees to bring the pad of the thumb in opposition to the lateral aspect of the second distal phalanx. The MCP joint extended to neutral, while the IP joint flexed 35 degrees. The second MCP joint extended 15 degrees, the PIP joint flexed to 55 degrees, and the DIP joint flexed to 35 degrees. The right hand performed the same motions as the left hand except for the abduction component of the thumb. The right thumb moved directly to the adduction component.[2] All ranges were the same as the left side. The other digits (four and five) remained relaxed in the

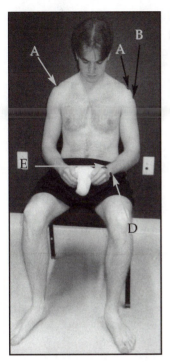

Figure 6-2. Grasping the sock: The subject grasped the sock with both hands to begin positioning the sock for donning. The key landmarks denoted by black dots are: A = acromion process; B = greater tuberosity of humerus; D = ulnar head (dorsal aspect); and E = radial styloid process (dorsal aspect)

resting position throughout the remainder of the task. The subject now had the sock grasped between the two hands.

From this two-jaw chuck grasp, the subject switched to a three-jaw chuck grasp bilaterally. Both thumbs abducted 5 degrees, moving the lateral aspect of the second distal phalanx in contact with the pads of both the second and third distal phalanges. The MCP joints of the third digit flexed to neutral, the PIP joints flexed to 85 degrees, and the DIP joints flexed to 35 degrees.[3-4] This positioned both hands so that the fingers were able to begin to gather the sock upward so that the three-jaw chuck ended just proximal to the toe part of the sock. This enabled the subject to pull the sock over the toes in the latter phase of the activity.

To gather the sock upward, the subject alternated with side-to-side motions. One wrist was extended 10 degrees, while the ipsilateral second and third MCP joints extended 10 degrees, then flexed back to neutral. As the MCP joint returned to neutral, the PIP joints flexed to 90 degrees and the DIP joints flexed to 45 degrees, pulling the more distal sock material into opposition with the pad of the thumb. At the same time, the wrist returned to its starting position of 5 degrees of extension.

Once this was completed, the activity alternated to the opposite upper extremity where the same motions were observed. This alternating activity continued until the digits had grasped the sock material just proximal to the toe of the sock (see Figure 6-2).

To achieve the horizontal adduction of both shoulder joints, the pectoralis major muscles worked concentrically. The brachialis muscles worked eccentrically to maintain the position of the elbow joints. The left pronators teres and quadratus worked concentrically to bring the left forearm into pronation. The right pronators worked eccentrically to maintain the position of the right forearm due to the influence of the extended position of the right wrist, causing more weight to fall on the lateral side of the forearm. This additional weight, as well as the influence of gravity, had a tendency to pull the forearm into supination. The bilateral wrist extensor muscles (extensors carpi radialis longus and brevis and carpi ulnaris) brought the wrists into their extended positions.[5-8]

The left pollicis abductors longus and brevis, acting concentrically, initiated the motion of the left thumb, followed by concentric contraction of the pollicis adductor to complete the motion. In addition, the extensors pollicis longus and brevis muscles contracted concentrically to extend the MCP joint and then the extensor pollicis longus reversed its activity (to eccentric contraction) to allow the IP joint to flex with the influence of gravity. By the end of this motion, the opponens pollicis muscle fired concentrically to help oppose the thumb to the second digit. The extensor digitorum muscle worked concentrically to extend the MCP joint of the second digit. The flexor digitorum profundus then worked concentrically to achieve the final flexed position of the PIP and DIP joints. The right finger muscles performed the same activities. The only difference was that the abductors of the right thumb did not fire, as no abduction occurred on the right side.[9-11]

As the subject switched to a three-jaw chuck, the abductors pollicis longus and brevis muscles of both hands were reactivated concentrically to reposition the thumb for this grasp. The flexor digitorum profundus muscle worked concentrically to flex the third digit. Following this, the adductor pollicis muscle worked concentrically to reestablish the opposition of the thumbs to the second and third digits.[12]

Next, the subject began the alternating motions to gather the sock upward. The extensors carpi radialii longus and brevis and carpi ulnaris muscles worked concentrically to extend the wrist. The extensor digitorum muscle worked concentrically to extend the MCP joints of the second and third digits. This muscle then worked eccentrically to return the MCP joints to neutral. The flexor digitorum profundus muscle worked concentrically to flex the more distal joints of the digits.

By the end of this maneuver, the wrist flexor muscles (flexors carpi radialis and carpi ulnaris) worked concentrically to flex the wrist back to its starting position in this phase. Once this activity had been completed, the muscles of the opposite extremity functioned in the same way to achieve the same motions.

Bringing the Sock to the Toes of the Foot

The next phase covered the motions from the grasping of the toe of the sock until the sock was brought to the toes of the right foot (Figure 6-3). The ending grasp was maintained by the digits during this entire phase. The initial forward movement of the upper extremities was brought about by forward flexion of the trunk and rotation to the right. Once the subject's hands had cleared the lap (just anterior to the knee joints), both shoulders were forward flexed to 95 degrees. The left shoulder was internally rotated an additional 10 to 15 degrees, while the right shoulder was maintained in its 45 degrees of internal rotation (Figure 6-4). Both elbow joints were fully extended and both forearms were pronated 5 to 10 degrees. The right wrist joint was extended 5 degrees, while the left wrist came to a neutral position. The subject had now brought the sock to the toes of the right foot.

The maintenance of the grasp of the sock was brought about by isometric contractions of the hand muscles described at the end of the last phase.[12-13] The initial forward movement of the upper extremities was brought about by trunk motion. As the subject's hands cleared the lap, the anterior deltoid and coracobrachialis muscles were activated concentrically to bring the shoulders into forward flexion. The left subscapularis muscle worked concentrically to internally rotate the left shoulder.[14-15] The triceps brachii and anconeus muscles worked concentrically to bring the elbows into full extension.[16-17] The pronators positioned the forearms in their 5 to 10 degrees of pronation. The right wrist was extended by the extensors carpi radialii longus and brevis and carpi ulnaris (working concentrically), while the left wrist was flexed to neutral by the left wrist extensors working eccentrically.

Placing the Sock Over the Heel and Lower Leg

The third phase covered the activity from placement of the sock at the toes to placement of the sock over the calcaneus of the right foot and lower leg (Figure 6-5). The grasp of the sock was maintained bilaterally, with only a slight loosening of the grasp noted to release the sock material as

Figure 6-3. Bringing the sock to the toes of the right foot. The key landmarks denoted by black dots are: A = acromion process; B = greater tuberosity of humerus; C = lateral epicondyle of humerus; H = ulnar styloid process (ulnar aspect); I = fifth MCP joint line (ulnar aspect); and J = olecranon process.

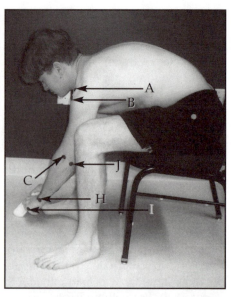

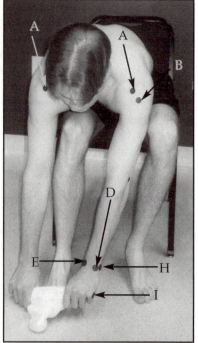

Figure 6-4. Anterior view of the sock being pulled over the toes of the right foot. The key landmarks denoted by black dots are: A = acromion process; B = greater tuberosity of humerus; D = ulnar head (dorsal aspect); E = radial styloid process (dorsal aspect); H = ulnar styloid process (ulnar aspect); and I = fifth MCP joint line (ulnar aspect).

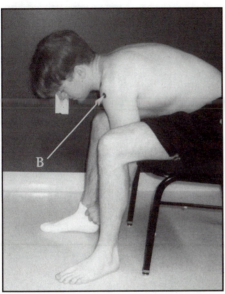

Figure 6-5. Placing the sock over the heel and lower leg of the right foot. The key landmark denoted by the black dots is B = greater tuberosity of humerus.

B

the sock was drawn upward over the foot. Simultaneously, the ankle joint was dorsiflexed to allow the sock to be pulled over the toes.

The position of the wrists and forearms was maintained during this time. The main motion came from the elbow and shoulder joints. The shoulder joints began to extend to pull the sock upward.

Simultaneously, the ankle joint was plantarflexed, returning the toes to the floor and lifting the heel off the floor (Figure 6-6). As the sock cleared the heel, the elbow joints began to flex. The shoulder joints came to lie in 90 degrees of flexion and the elbow joints in 15 degrees of flexion by the end of this phase, at which time the sock was in position on the foot and lower leg of the subject (see Figure 6-5).

Muscular activity of the digits was primarily isometric in nature, with minimal change in contraction as the grasp was loosened slightly to release the sock material. At that time, there was a momentary eccentric contraction of the muscles, followed by a concentric contraction and then a return to isometric contraction.

The muscles of the wrist and forearms maintained an isometric contraction to keep these body parts positioned.[18] The posterior deltoid and latissimus dorsi muscles worked concentrically to move the shoulders into extension. The brachialis muscles worked concentrically to flex the elbows.

Figure 6-6. Placing the sock over the heel of the right foot: The ankle joint is plantarflexed. The key landmarks denoted by black dots are: A = acromion process; B = greater tuberosity of humerus; D = ulnar head (dorsal aspect); E = radial styloid process (dorsal aspect); and G = first MCP joint line.

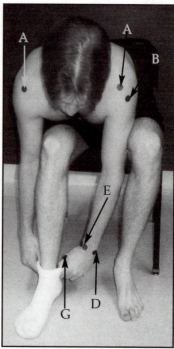

RETURN OF THE SUBJECT TO THE STARTING POSITION

The final phase covered the return of the subject to the initial upright seated position. Once the sock was in place, the grasp was released bilaterally by extension of the joints of the second and third digits and abduction and extension of the joints of the thumb. Only 2 to 3 degrees of motion were needed to accomplish this release. The elbow and shoulder joints were maintained in their previous phase ending positions, while the trunk was brought back to an upright position (Figure 6-7). The trunk was extended and rotated to the left until the neutral position was achieved. The elbow and shoulder joints, as well as the more distal joints of the upper extremity, were then returned to their starting positions on the subject's lap. The subject was now ready to begin the process again and don the left sock. The analysis of the left upper extremity was similar to that of the right upper extremity. The main difference was the reversal of the upper extremity usage and rotation of the trunk to the left.

To release the grasp on the sock, the extensor digitorum muscle acted concentrically to extend the joints of the second and third digit.

Bringing the Sock to the Toes of the Foot

- Primarily flexion of shoulder and left wrist joints.

- Extension of elbow and right wrist joints.

- Pronation of radioulnar joints.

- Primarily concentric muscular activity.

- Digits are maintaining their position via isometric muscular contraction.

Placing the Sock Over the Heel and Lower Leg

- Primarily shoulder extension and elbow flexion via concentric muscular contractions.

- All other joints are maintaining their positions via isometric muscular activity.

Return of the Subject to the Starting Position

- Both shoulder joints continue in extension.

- Both elbow joints continue in flexion.

- Primarily eccentric muscular activity.

- Digits in minimal extension and abduction.

- Primarily concentric muscular activity.

CLINICAL APPLICATION AND DISCUSSION QUESTIONS

This analysis has presented one method of donning ankle-length socks. Think about your own method of dressing. How does your method compare to that presented in this chapter?

How would the upper extremity activity change if the foot was brought toward the upper extremity? How would it change if the subject stood and propped the foot on a bed or chair? How would the muscular analysis change if a calf-length sock were used? How would the donning of pantyhose or stockings change this analysis? How would this compare to donning post-surgical compression hose?

Although this analysis focused on upper extremity usage, think about the activity of the trunk and lower extremities. Which motions are key to the completion of this task? What muscles are the prime movers for those motions? Compare your findings for the lower extremities to the analysis presented in Chapter 11.

What assistive devices could be used in an activity such as this? How would these devices benefit the person performing the activity?

Finally, make a list of muscles that could be substituted for the prime movers in this analysis. Compare your substitutions with those listed in Chart 1 in Appendix A.

REFERENCES

1.   Atkeson CG. Learning arm kinematics and dynamics. *Annu Rev Neurosci.* 1989;12:157-183.

2.   Buchholz B, Armstrong TJ. A kinematic model of the human hand to evaluate its prehensile abilities. *J Biomech.* 1992;25:149-162.

3.   Jones LA. The assessment of hand function: a critical review of techniques. *J Hand Surg Am.* 1989;14:221-228.

4.   Landsmeer JMF. Power grip and precision handling. *Ann Rheum Dis.* 1962;21:164-170.

5.   Schenkman M, DeCartaya VR. Kinesiology of the shoulder complex. *J Orthop Sports Phys Ther.* 1987;8:438-450.

6.   Basmajian JV, Latif A. Integrated actions and functions of the chief flexors of the elbow: a detailed electromyographic analysis. *J Bone Joint Surg Am.* 1957;39:1106-1118.

7.   Pauly JE, Rushing JL, Scheving LE. An electromyographic study of some muscles crossing the elbow joint. *Anat Rec.* 1967;159:47-53.

8.   Erdman AG, Mayfield JK, Dorman F, Wallrich M, Dahlof W. Kinematic and kinetic analysis of the human wrist by stereoscopic instrumentation. *J Biomech Eng.* 1979;101:124-133.

9.   An KN, Chao EY, Cooney WP, Linscheid RI. Tendon excursion and moment arm of index finger muscles. *J Biomech.* 1983;16:419-426.

10. Brand PW, Cranor KC, Ellis JC. Tendon and pulleys at the metacarpophalangeal joint of a finger. *J Bone Joint Surg Am.* 1975;57:779-784.

11. Sunderland S. Actions of the extensor digitorum communis, interosseous, and lumbrical muscles. *American Journal of Anatomy.* 1945;77:189-194.

12. Long C, Conrad PW, Hall EA, Furler SL. Intrinsic-extrinsic muscle control of the hand in power grip and precision handling: an electromyographic study. *J Bone Joint Surg Br.* 1970;52:853-867.

13. Chao EY, Opgrande JD, Axmear FE. Three-dimensional force analysis of finger joints in selected isometric hand functions. *J Biomech.* 1976;9:387-396.

14. Blakely RL, Palmer ML. Analysis of rotation accompanying shoulder flexion. *Phys Ther.* 1984;64:1214-1216.

15. Kronberg M, Nemeth G, Brostrom L. Muscle activity and coordination in the normal shoulder. *Clin Orthop.* 1990;257:76-85.

16. Little AD, Lehmkuhl D. Elbow extension force measured in three positions. *Phys Ther.* 1966;46:7-17.

17. Basmajian JV, Griffin WR. Function of anconeus muscle: an electromyographic study. *J Bone Joint Surg Am.* 1972;54:1712-1714.

18. Wadsworth CT. Clinical anatomy and mechanics of the wrist and hand. *J Orthop Sports Phys Ther.* 1983;4:206-216.

SUGGESTED READINGS

An KN, Chao EY, Cooney WP, Linscheid RI. Normative model of human hand for biomechanical analysis. *J Biomech.* 1979;12:775-788.

An KN, Hui FC, Morrey BF, Linscheid RI, Chao EY. Muscles across the elbow joint: a biomechanical analysis. *J Biomech.* 1981;14:659-669.

Bechtol C. Biomechanics of the shoulder. *Clin Orthop.* 1980;146:37-41.

Brumfield RH, Champoux JA. A biomechanical study of normal functional wrist motion. *Clin Orthop.* 1979;187:23-25.

Culham E, Peat M. Functional anatomy of the shoulder complex. *J Orthop Sports Phys Ther.* 1993;18:342-350.

Engin AE. On the biomechanics of the shoulder complex. *J Biomech.* 1980;13:575-590.

Griffin JW. Differences in elbow flexion torque measured concentrically, eccentrically, and isometrically. *Phys Ther.* 1987;67:1205-1208.

Hagberg M. Electromyographic signs of shoulder muscular fatigue in two elevated arm positions. *Am J Phys Med Rehabil.* 1981;60:111-121.

Herberts P, Kadefors R, Broman H. Arm positioning in manual tasks—an electromyographic study of localized muscle fatigue. *Ergonomics.* 1980;23:655-665.

Ishizuki M. Functional anatomy of the elbow joint and three-dimensional quantitative analysis of the elbow joint. *Journal of the Japanese Orthopedic Association.* 1979;53:986-989.

Perry T. Normal upper extremity kinesiology. *Phys Ther.* 1978;58:165-178.

Ryu J, Cooney WP, Askew LJ, An KN, Chao EYS. Functional ranges of motion of the wrist joint. *J Hand Surg Am.* 1991;16:409-419.

Singh M, Karpovich PV. Isotonic and isometric forces of forearm flexors and extensors. *J Appl Physiol.* 1966;21:1435-1437.

Taylor CL, Blaschke AC. A method for kinematic analysis of the shoulder, arm, and hand complex. *Ann N Y Acad Sci.* 1951;51:1251-1265.

Taylor CL, Schwarz RJ. The anatomy and mechanics of the human hand. *Artificial Limbs.* 1955;2:22-34.

Chapter 7

Tying Shoelaces

INTRODUCTION AND SET-UP

Think for a moment about tying your shoelaces. Do you tie each shoe after putting it on? Do you put on both shoes and then tie both shoelaces? When tying your shoelaces, do you cross the right lace over the left lace or vice versa? Do you make two loops simultaneously before you make the final knot? Do you sit or stand to tie your shoes? Do you elevate your foot, or do you leave your foot on the floor? Can you visualize your technique without actually tying your shoes?

Most individuals tie their shoes everyday without even thinking about it. This is an activity that gets repeated numerous times throughout one's lifetime. In observing a group of individuals tying their shoes, a variety of techniques would be seen. This particular analysis focused on the motions of the upper extremities. It started with the subject seated in a chair in which the seat was 18 inches from the ground. The left hip and knee joints were fully flexed to place the sole of the shoe on the seat of the chair. The trunk was slightly flexed and rotated to the left. The arms were positioned on either side of the left knee. The right hand was holding one shoelace (dark in color for the sake of clarity in this analysis), and the left hand was holding the other shoelace (light in color). Extra long shoelaces were used for this activity to enable the reader to have a better visualization of the technique used. A three-jaw chuck, pad-to-pad grip (first three digits) was used to hold the lace on the right side. The tips of the other two digits were resting against the lace. A lateral prehension-type grip was used to hold the lace on the left side, with the thumb in opposition to the radial aspect of the index finger (Figure 7-1).

In this starting position, the left shoulder joint was flexed 40 degrees, abducted 33 degrees, and internally rotated 5 degrees. The right shoulder joint was flexed 47 degrees and internally rotated 5 degrees.

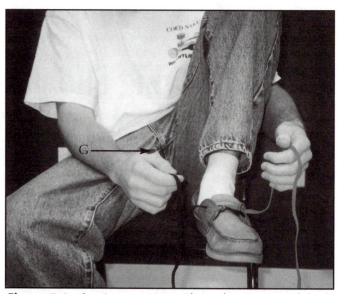

Figure 7-1. Starting position: The subject grasped both shoelaces. There was a three-jaw chuck grip on the right side and a lateral prehension grip on the left side. The key landmark denoted by the black dot is G = first MCP joint line.

The left elbow joint was flexed 58 degrees, while the right elbow was flexed 61 degrees. The forearms were in neutral, as were the wrist joints in terms of flexion and extension. Both wrist joints were radially deviated 3 degrees.

The right second through fifth digits were in flexion, while the thumb was opposed to digits two and three. The MCP joints of the left second through fifth digits were flexed 31, 39, 34, and 49 degrees, respectively; those of the right hand were flexed 40, 45, 44, and 45 degrees, respectively. The PIP joints of the left hand were flexed 54, 65, 58, and 54 degrees, respectively; those of the right hand were flexed 38, 55, 53, and 35 degrees, respectively. Finally, the DIP joints of the left hand were flexed 35, 33, 20, and 35 degrees, respectively; those of the right hand were flexed 30, 41, 25, and 30 degrees, respectively.

From this starting position, the activity was divided into three main phases: the first phase described the initiation of tying the bow; the second phase, completion of tying the bow; and the third phase, tightening and securing the bow.

INITIATION OF TYING THE BOW

From the described starting position, the subject began to tie the shoelace of the left shoe. The right index finger extended to neutral at the MCP joint to release the grip on the lace.[1-4] The right index finger was then flexed 30 degrees at the MCP joint to reposition it to grip both laces. The left index finger was extended to neutral at the MCP joint to release its grip on the lace. The light-colored lace was pushed under the dark-colored lace with the left index finger through 49 degrees of flexion of its MCP joint (Figure 7-2). The left thumb extended and abducted to neutral at its CMC joint. The IP joint of the left thumb fully flexed until it passed beneath the dark lace. Next, the left thumb was consecutively extended fully at the IP, MCP, and CMC joints to catch the light lace on its fingernail and draw it all the way through.[5-6] The MCP joint of the left index finger extended to neutral. The left thumb was then opposed to the index finger to pinch the lace between these two fingers. During this action, the index finger abducted 1 degree, while the thumb opposed it.

To pull the shoe laces tight, both shoulder joints remained flexed. The left shoulder joint abducted an additional degree, while the right shoulder abducted 5 degrees. The left shoulder joint remained in its internally rotated position. The right shoulder joint externally rotated 2 to 3 degrees. The left elbow joint flexed an additional 6 degrees; the right elbow, an additional ½ degree. The right forearm, bringing the light lace behind the dark lace, supinated 47 degrees. The left side remained in neutral. The right wrist joint remained in neutral, while the left wrist joint flexed 40 degrees. The radial deviation of the left side increased from 3 to 20 degrees. The radial deviation of the right wrist joint remained the same (Figure 7-3).

The left second through fifth digits were mainly flexed, with the thumb opposed to the second digit. The MCP joints of digits two through five were flexed 49, 50, 63, and 57 degrees, respectively. Those of the right side were flexed 30, 52, 40, and 39 degrees, respectively. The left PIP joints were flexed 63, 90, 85, and 63 degrees, respectively, while the right PIP joints were flexed 74, 91, 98, and 75 degrees, respectively. The left DIP joints were flexed 51, 58, 44, and 58 degrees, respectively, while the right DIP joints were flexed 44, 73, 70, and 70 degrees, respectively. In general, these goniometric measurements represented an increase in the amount of flexion that had occurred from the starting to the end position of this phase. However, the measurements of the right MCP joints of the second, fourth, and fifth digits represented a decrease in flexion. This difference was due to the positioning of those digits to manipulate the shoelaces as the task proceeded. By the end of this phase, the subject was using a power grip on the right side and a two-jaw chuck on the left side (Figure 7-3).

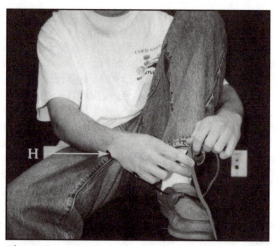

Figure 7-2. Initiation of tying the bow: The subject had started to cross the light-colored lace under the dark-colored lace. The key landmark denoted by the black dot is H = ulnar styloid process (ulnar aspect).

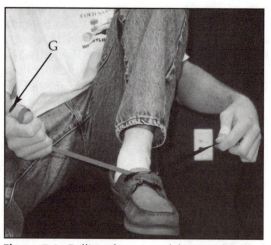

Figure 7-3. Pulling the crossed laces tight: The subject used a power grip on the right side and a two-jaw chuck on the left. The key landmark denoted by the black dot is G = first MCP joint line.

COMPLETION OF TYING THE BOW

At this point in the activity, the subject began the second phase: completion of tying the bow. There was a return to neutral by pronation of the right forearm and extension of the left wrist. The shoelaces were balanced on the sides of the index fingers to allow the thumbs to extend at the CMC joints. The MCP joints of the third fingers were extended, while the PIP and DIP joints were flexed and then extended to reach past the shoelaces. Next, the MCP joints were flexed to pull each shoe lace forward until they met. The shoelaces were now forming two loops. The CMC and MCP joints of both thumbs were flexed until they grasped each of the loops in a three-jaw chuck[7-8] (Figure 7-4).

The dark lace was crossed behind the light lace (Figure 7-5) by flexing and ulnarly deviating both wrist joints. Next, the MCP joint of the right index finger was extended in preparation for holding both loops. To secure a pad-to-pad grip with the right thumb, the MCP joint was flexed again. The MCP joint of the left index finger extended until it passed beyond the light loop. The MCP joint was then extended to push the light loop beneath the cross loops. Supination of the left forearm assisted this maneuver. Next, the left thumb was extended at the CMC joint in preparation for the next movement of the light loop. All the joints of the left thumb were flexed to position the thumb under the light loop. The MCP and IP joints of the left thumb then extended, while the CMC joint continued to flex and adduct to catch the light loop in a pad-to-side grip between the left thumb and the index finger.

TIGHTENING AND SECURING THE BOW

To pull the bow tight, the forearms were supinated, and the wrist and elbow joints were extended. The task was completed: the left shoelace had been tied. In this ending position, both shoulder joints were flexed. The left shoulder joint was flexed 35 degrees, and the right, 36 degrees. In addition, the left shoulder was abducted 32 degrees and internally rotated 5 degrees. The right shoulder was in neutral. Both elbow joints were flexed (left at 70 degrees and right at 59 degrees). The right forearm was pronated 6 degrees; the left was in neutral. Both wrist joints were in neutral (Figure 7-6).

The digits of the hand were primarily flexed, with the thumb opposed to the second digit on the right side and the thumb opposed to the second and third digit on the left side. On the left side, the thumb was flexed 45 degrees at the MCP joint and extended 5 degrees at the IP joint.

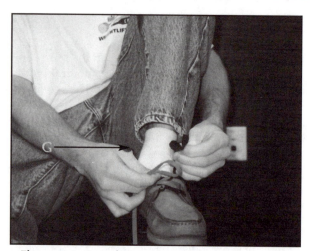

Figure 7-4. Completion of tying the bow: The subject used a three-jaw chuck bilaterally to grasp the loops of the bow. The key landmark denoted by the black dot is G = first MCP joint line.

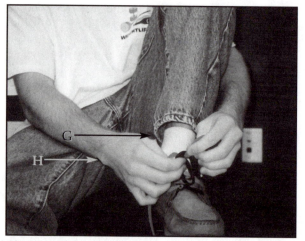

Figure 7-5. Completion of tying the bow: The subject crossed the dark lace behind the light lace to complete the bow. The key landmarks denoted by black dots are: G = first MCP joint line and H = ulnar styloid process (ulnar aspect).

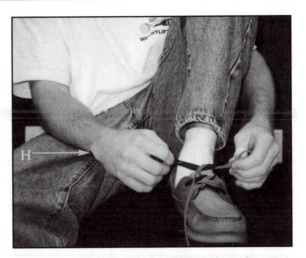

Figure 7-6. Tightening the bow: The subject began to tighten the bow by pulling on the loops of the laces. The key landmark denoted by the black dot is H = ulnar styloid process (ulnar aspect).

On the right side, the thumb was flexed 35 degrees at the MCP joint and 20 degrees at the IP joint. On the left side, there was 48, 63, 53, and 35 degrees of flexion at the MCP joints of the second through fifth digits. On the right side, there was 30, 35, 23, and 20 degrees of flexion, respectively. The left PIP joints were in 65, 73, 85, and 73 degrees of flexion, respectively; the right, 66, 66, 79, and 70 degrees, respectively. The left DIP joints were in 46, 43, 35, and 63 degrees of flexion, respectively; the right, 43, 48, 48, and 65 degrees, respectively.

During this entire activity, the shoulder joints were maintained in their flexed position by isometric contractions of anterior deltoid and coracobrachialis muscles. Concentric contractions of the middle deltoid and supraspinatus muscles caused the abduction bilaterally. The subscapularis, pectoralis major, latissimus dorsi, and teres major muscles worked concentrically on the left to bring about internal rotation. On the right side, the infraspinatus and teres minor muscles worked concentrically to produce the external rotation.[9-13] The biceps brachii worked concentrically to produce the additional flexion of both elbow joints. The triceps and anconeus muscles worked eccentrically to assist with placement of the elbow joints during this time. At times, these elbow muscles worked isometrically to maintain the position of the elbow joints while the hands were manipulating the shoelaces.[14-15]

The right forearm was supinated by concentric activity of the supinators. The left forearm was maintained in its neutral position through synergistic activity of the supinators and pronators. The right wrist joint was held in neutral by synergistic activity of the flexors carpi ulnaris and radialis and extensors carpi ulnaris and radialii longus and brevis muscles. The flexors worked concentrically on the left to bring about the flexion of the left wrist joint. However, the flexor carpi radialis and the extensor carpi radialii longus and brevis exerted a greater influence due to the radial deviation of both wrists. There may have been activity of the palmaris longus muscle in individuals who have this muscle. The use of this muscle would assist in enhancing the cupping effect of the palm. In turn, this cupping effect would support the positioning of the digits for function. The wrist extensors worked concentrically when extension of the wrist was needed. These changes were important to maintain a good length-tension relationship for the long finger muscles to work effectively.[16-17] As with the shoulder and elbow musculature, the muscles of the forearm and wrist worked isometrically to hold the forearm and wrist positions when needed.

The finger muscles demonstrated primarily isometric activity to maintain a grasp on the shoelaces. However, there was an interplay between the flexors and extensors and the abductors and adductors of the thumb to manipulate the shoes laces. The flexors digitorum superficialis and profundus and the extensors digitorum, indicis, and digiti minimi were the primary muscles involved in the activity of digits two through five. The adductor pollicis, abductors pollicis longus and brevis, and the opponens pollicis were the primary muscles moving the thumb. In addition, the first dorsal interosseous muscle was important for the abduction motion of the second digit. A concentric contraction of this muscle caused the abduction to occur.[4,18-19]

SUMMARY

Key Anatomical Landmarks for Shoelace Analysis

Shoulder Complex:	Greater tuberosity of humerus
	Acromion process (dorsal aspect)
Elbow and Forearm Complex:	Lateral epicondyle of humerus
	Radial styloid process (dorsal aspect)
	Radial styloid process (radial aspect)
	Ulnar head (dorsal aspect)
	Ulnar styloid process (ulnar aspect)

Wrist and Hand Complex:	Base of first MCP (radial and palmar aspects)
	Base of second MCP (dorsal aspect)
	Base of fifth MCP (dorsal aspect)
	First MCP joint line (palmar aspect)
	Second MCP joint line (radial aspect)
	Fifth MCP joint line (ulnar aspect)
	First IP joint line (palmar aspect)
	Second PIP joint line (radial aspect)
	Fifth PIP joint line (ulnar aspect)
	Second DIP joint line (radial aspect)
	Fifth DIP joint line (ulnar aspect)

Major Phases for Shoelace Analysis

Starting Position

- Position of subject

- Position of the shoelace

Initiation of Tying the Bow

Completion of Tying the Bow

Tightening and Securing the Bow

Upper Extremity Joint Motions and Muscular Activity: Tying Shoelaces

Introduction and Set-Up

- Primarily flexion of the proximal and distal joints.

- Radioulnar joints in neutral.

- Radial deviation of the wrist joints.

Initiation of Tying the Bow

- Primarily maintenance of position of shoulder and left radioulnar joints.

- Flexion of elbow and left wrist joints.

- Supination of right radioulnar joint.

- Digits underwent extension, flexion, abduction, and opposition.

- Primarily isometric and concentric muscular activity.

Completion of Tying the Bow

- Supination of left radioulnar joint and pronation of right radioulnar joint.

- Extension of left wrist joint and flexion of right wrist joint.

- Primarily extension and flexion of digits.

- Primarily concentric and eccentric muscular activity.

Tightening and Securing the Bow

- Shoulder and left radioulnar joints maintaining their positions via isometric muscular activity.

- Flexion of left elbow joint and extension of right elbow joint.

- Extension of wrist joints and pronation of right radioulnar joint.

- Primarily concentric and eccentric muscular activity.

- Digits are maintaining their positions via isometric muscular activity.

CLINICAL APPLICATION AND DISCUSSION QUESTIONS

Return to the beginning of this chapter and review the questions that introduced it. Close your eyes. Can you picture how you do this activity? Which shoe do you tie first? Do you make a double loop with the laces and intertwine them to form the bow? Do you form one loop and then bring the other lace through it to form the bow? Could you do this activity one-handed? Try it and see. How does this compare to using two hands?

Now think about the convenience of elastic shoelaces or Velcro closures for those individuals who have lost the ability to tie their laces. How does the use of Velcro closures compare to tying laces?

Compare this activity analysis to wrapping a present with a fancy bow or wrapping a package with a string.

Generate a list of the muscles that could be substituted for the prime movers presented in this analysis. Compare your list to Chart 1 in Appendix A.

REFERENCES

1. An KN, Chao EY, Cooney WP, Linscheid RI. Normative model of human hand for biomechanical analysis. *J Biomech.* 1979;12:775-788.

2. Buchholz B, Armstrong TJ. A kinematic model of the human hand to evaluate its prehensile abilities. *J Biomech.* 1992;25:149-162.

3. Jones LA. The assessment of hand function: a critical review of techniques. *J Hand Surg Am.* 1989;14;221-228.

4. Landsmeer JMF. Power grip and precision handling. *Ann Rheum Dis.* 1962;21:164-170.

5. Barmakian JT. Anatomy of the joints of the thumb. *Hand Clin.* 1992;8:683-691.

6. Iamdea T, An K, Cooney WP. Functional anatomy and biomechanics of the thumb. *Hand Clin.* 1992;8:9-15.

7. Craig SM. Anatomy of the joints of the fingers. *Hand Clin.* 1992;8:693-700.

8. Landsmeer JMF. Anatomical and functional investigations on the articulation of the human fingers. *Acta Anat (Basel).* 1955;25, suppl 24.

9. DeLuca CJ, Forrest WJ. Force analysis of individual muscles acting simultaneously on the shoulder joint during isometric abduction. *J Biomech.* 1973;6:385-393.

10. Hart DL, Carmicheal SW. Biomechanics of the shoulder. *J Orthop Sports Phys Ther.* 1985;16:229-278.

11. Howell SM, Imoberseg AM, Seger DH, Marone PJ. Clarification of the role of the supraspinatus muscle in shoulder function. *J Bone Joint Surg Am.* 1985;68:398-404.

12. Jarp Y. Activation of the rotator cuff in generating isometric shoulder rotation torque. *Am J Sports Med.* 1996;24:477-485.

13. Saha AK. Dynamic stability of the glenohumeral joint. *Acta Orthop Scand.* 1971;42:491-505.

14. Currier DP. Maximal isometric tension of the elbow extensors at varied positions. *Phys Ther.* 1972;52:1043-1049.

15. Pauly JE, Rushing RJ, Scheving LE. An electromyographic study of some muscles crossing the elbow joint. *Anat Rec.* 1967;159:47-53.

16. Volz RG, Lieb M, Benjamin J. Biomechanics of the wrist. *Clin Orthop.* 1980;149: 112-117.
17. Wadsworth CT. Clinical anatomy and mechanics of the wrist and hand. *J Orthop Sports Phys Ther.* 1983;4:206-216.
18. Chao EY, Opgrande JD, Axmear FE. Three-dimensional force analysis of finger joints in selected isometric hand functions. *J Biomech.* 1976;9:387-396.
19. Long C, Conrad PW, Hall EA, Furler SL. Intrinsic-extrinsic muscle control of the hand in power grip and precision handling: an electromyographic study. *J Bone Joint Surg Br.* 1970;52:853-867.

SUGGESTED READINGS

An KN, Hui FC, Morrey BF, Linscheid RL, Chao EY. Muscles across the elbow joint: a biomechanical analysis. *J Biomech.* 1981;14:659-669.

Atkeson CG. Learning arm kinematics and dynamics. *Annu Rev Neurosci.* 1989;12:157-183.

Bechtol C. Biomechanics of the shoulder. *Clin Orthop.* 1980;146:37-41.

Brumfield RH, Champoux JA. A biomechanical study of normal functional wrist motion. *Clin Orthop.* 1979;187:23-25.

Carmichael SW, Hart DL. Anatomy of the shoulder joint. *J Orthop Sports Phys Ther.* 1985;6:225-228.

Engen TJ, Spencer WA. Method of kinematic study of normal upper extremity movements. *Arch Phys Med Rehabil.* 1968;49:9-11.

Hagberg M. Electromyographic signs of shoulder muscular fatigue in two elevated arm positions. *Am J Phys Med Rehabil.* 1981;60:111-121.

Hankinson JL. Tying a shoelace one-handed. *Physiother.* 1984;70:200.

Herberts P, Kadefors R, Broman H. Arm positioning in manual tasks—an electromyographic study of localized muscle fatigue. *Ergonomics.* 1980;23:655-665.

Hills RE. Tying a shoelace one-handed. *Physiother.* 1984;70:395.

Singh M, Karpovich PV. Isotonic and isometric forces of forearm flexors and extensors. *J Appl Physiol.* 1966;21:1435-1437.

Stroyan M, Wilk KE. The functional anatomy of the elbow complex. *J Orthop Sports Phys Ther.*1993;17:279-288.

Taylor CL, Schwarz RJ. The anatomy and mechanics of the human hand. *Artificial Limbs.* 1955;2:22-34.

Chapter 8

Stirring a Batter

INTRODUCTION AND SET-UP

The upper extremities are key components when preparing a cake batter. This analysis focused on the motions and muscular activity of the upper extremities. The subject was standing in front of the work surface. All the ingredients for the cake batter were in the mixing bowl. The right hand was grasping a mixing spoon held in the bowl. A modified cylindrical grip was used to grasp the spoon. The left upper extremity was used to stabilize the mixing bowl by positioning the bowl between the forearm and the trunk. The left hand was cupped around the bowl. From this starting position, the subject began to stir the batter ingredients (Figure 8-1).

The right glenohumeral joint was in 8 degrees of abduction, and the elbow joint was in 88 degrees of flexion at the above starting position. The sternoclavicular and acromioclavicular joints were protracted. The radioulnar joints were pronated 84 degrees. The wrist joints were in 45 degrees of flexion and 10 degrees of ulnar deviation. The first CMC joint was in 14 degrees of flexion and 32 degrees of abduction. The first MCP joint was flexed 25 degrees, and the IP joint was hyperextended 15 degrees. The second MCP joint was flexed 38 degrees, while the third through fifth MCP joints were flexed 64, 92, and 95 degrees, respectively. The second PIP joint was extended. The third through the fifth PIP joints were flexed 90, 95, and 90 degrees, respectively. The second through fifth DIP joints were flexed 45, 90, 90, and 90 degrees, respectively (Figure 8-2).

STIRRING THE BATTER—RIGHT UPPER EXTREMITY

As the subject began to stir the batter, the glenohumeral joint abducted an additional 5 degrees, extended 5 degrees, and laterally rotated 5

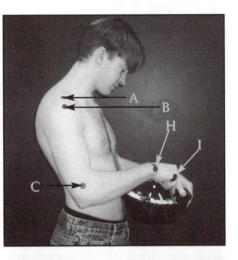

Figure 8-1. Starting position: The subject used a modified cylindrical grip to grasp the spoon. The key landmarks denoted by black dots are: A = acromion process; B = greater tuberosity of humerus; C = lateral epicondyle; H = ulnar styloid process (ulnar aspect); and I = fifth MCP joint line (ulnar aspect).

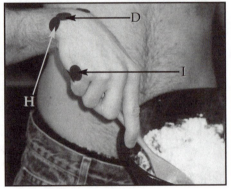

Figure 8-2. Close-up view of the right hand's grasp on the spoon. The key landmarks denoted by black dots are: D = ulnar head (dorsal aspect); H = ulnar styloid process (ulnar aspect); and I = fifth MCP joint line (ulnar aspect).

degrees. This was followed by the reverse motions of adduction, flexion, and medial rotation for the same amount of motion.[1-2] Essentially, the subject was performing a modified circumduction of the right upper extremity (Figures 8-3 and 8-4). The elbow joint flexed an additional 5 degrees, while the glenohumeral joint was abducting, extending, and laterally rotating. The motion was then reversed as the activity of the glenohumeral joint was reversed. The radioulnar joints remained in pronation. The wrist joint flexed an additional 5 to 10 degrees and maintained its ulnarly deviated position. The finger joints maintained their grip on the spoon as the activity continued. As the subject continued to stir the ingredients, the above motions were repeated by the right upper extremity.

The primary muscular activity of the right upper extremity involved in this ADL was concentric in nature. The serratus anterior and trapezius

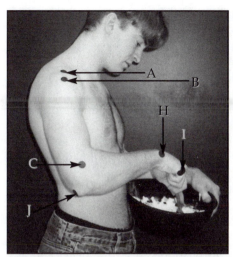

Figure 8-3. Stirring the batter with the right upper extremity. Subject used a modified circumduction to complete the task. The key landmarks denoted by black dots are: A = acromion process; B = greater tuberosity of humerus; C = lateral epicondyle; H = ulnar styloid process (ulnar aspect); I = fifth MCP joint line (ulnar aspect); and J = olecranon process.

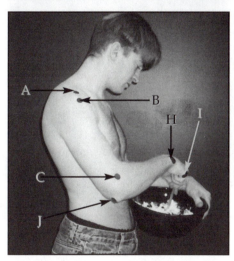

Figure 8-4. Stirring the batter with the right upper extremity. Completion of the circumduction to stir the batter. The key landmarks denoted by black dots are: A = acromion process; B = greater tuberosity of humerus; C = lateral epicondyle; H = ulnar styloid process (ulnar aspect); I = fifth MCP joint line (ulnar aspect); and J = olecranon process.

(upper and lower fibers) produced the abduction of the glenohumeral joint.[3] The pectoralis major, latissimus dorsi, and teres major muscles produced the adduction and medial rotation.[4-5] The deltoid muscle produced the flexion and extension motions, as well as the abduction component. In addition, the teres major muscle contributed to the extension motion. The subscapularis muscle produced the lateral rotation. These muscles worked synergistically to control the motions needed to stir the batter ingredients.[6-9]

The biceps brachii and the brachialis muscles worked concentrically and eccentrically to control the flexion and extension of the elbow joint.[10-12] The supinator and the pronators quadratus and teres rotated back and forth to control and maintain the position of the forearm.[13] The same was true for the muscles controlling the wrist joint. The flexors carpi radialis and ulnaris, the extensors carpi radialis longus and brevis, and the ulnaris muscles alternated between concentric and eccentric contractions. However, the flexors first worked concentrically and independently to produce the additional wrist flexion.[14-15]

The muscles of the fingers acted isometrically to maintain their grip on the spoon and overcome the resistance of the batter. These muscles included the extensors pollicis longus and brevis, the abductors pollicis longus and brevis, and the flexors pollicis longus and brevis. Initially, the flexor digitorum profundus was active to secure the grip of the spoon. The flexor digitorum superficialis then took over to maintain the grip during the mixing action. In addition, the lumbricals and the interossei muscles were active to maintain the MCP joint positions.[16-20]

STABILIZING THE BOWL—LEFT UPPER EXTREMITY

The left upper extremity was used as a stabilizing force in this activity[21] (Figure 8-5). The glenohumeral joint was abducted 12 degrees, extended 3 to 5 degrees, and medially rotated 5 degrees. The sternoclavicular and acromioclavicular joints were protracted. The elbow joint was in 60 degrees of flexion. The radioulnar joints were in the neutral position. The wrist joint was flexed 40 degrees. The finger joints were flexed as follows: the first CMC joint was flexed 24 degrees; the MCP joint, 35 degrees; and the IP joint, 24 degrees. The second through fifth MCP joints were flexed 40, 38, 35, and 30 degrees, respectively. The second through fifth PIP joints were extended. The second through fifth DIP joints were flexed 10, 10, 12, and 12 degrees, respectively. These positions of the joints of the left upper extremity remained constant throughout the activity.

In contrast to the right upper extremity, the primary muscle activity of the left upper extremity was isometric once the bowl had been stabilized. The serratus anterior, trapezius, pectoralis major, latissimus dorsi, teres major, and posterior deltoid muscles were active at the glenohumeral joint.[1,6-8,22-25] The biceps brachii, brachialis, and brachioradialis muscles were active at the elbow joint.[9-11]

Even though the radioulnar joints were maintained in a neutral position, there was a tendency toward supination as stabilization was maintained; the biceps brachii and the supinator muscles provided this stabilization.[12]

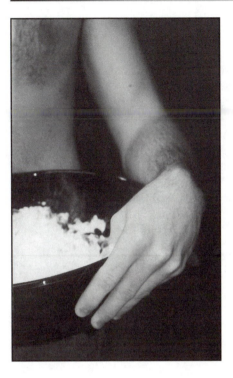

Figure 8-5. Close-up view of the left hand stabilizing the mixing bowl.

The flexors carpi radialis and ulnaris muscles further contributed to this stabilization by maintaining the wrist joint in its position.[13-14]

Finally, the finger joints were maintained in their position by the same muscles cited for the right upper extremity. The main difference was the amount of flexion in each finger. In addition, the abductors pollicis longus and brevis muscles were not needed in the left hand to provide stabilization of the mixing bowl.[15-19]

SUMMARY

Key Anatomical Landmarks for Stirring Analysis

Shoulder Complex: Greater tuberosity of humerus
                     Acromion process (dorsal aspect)

Elbow and Forearm   Lateral epicondyle of humerus
Complex: Radial styloid process (dorsal aspect)
                     Radial styloid process (radial aspect)

Ulnar head (dorsal aspect)
Ulnar styloid process (ulnar aspect)

Wrist and Hand
Complex:

Base of first MCP (radial and palmar aspects)
Base of second MCP (dorsal aspect)
Base of fifth MCP (dorsal aspect)
First MCP joint line (palmar aspect)
Second MCP joint line (radial aspect)
Fifth MCP joint line (ulnar aspect)
First IP joint line (palmar aspect)
Second PIP joint line (radial aspect)
Fifth PIP joint line (ulnar aspect)
Second DIP joint line (radial aspect)
Fifth DIP joint line (ulnar aspect)

Major Phases for Stirring Analysis

Starting Position

• Position of subject

• Height of work surface

• Position of mixing bowl

Stirring the Batter—Right Upper Extremity

Stabilizing the Bowl—Left Upper Extremity

Upper Extremity Joint Motions and Muscular Activity: Stirring a Batter

Introduction and Set-Up

• Shoulders in abduction.

• Left radioulnar joint in neutral and right radioulnar joint in pronation.

• Primarily flexion of distal joints.

Stirring a Batter—Right Upper Extremity

• Shoulder moving from abduction, extension, and external rotation to adduction, flexion, and internal rotation.

- Elbow moving from flexion to extension.

- Wrist in flexion.

- Radioulnar joints and digits maintaining their positions.

- Primarily concentric muscular activity proximally.

- Isometric muscular activity distally.

Stabilizing the Bowl—Left Upper Extremity
- All joints maintained their starting positions throughout the activity via isometric muscular activity.

CLINICAL APPLICATION AND DISCUSSION QUESTIONS

Obviously, this muscular analysis would change if the subject used an electric mixer to stir the batter. The other factors that would alter this analysis include the height of the working surface, the distance between the subject and the mixing bowl, and the consistency of the batter ingredients.

Describe the grip a subject would use on an electric hand-held mixer. How is it different from the grip used on a spoon? What effect will the vibrations generated by the electric mixer have on the muscular activity of the upper extremity?

What other ways could the mixing bowl be stabilized if the subject had use of one upper extremity only?

Compile a list of muscles that could be substituted for the prime movers in this analysis. Compare your suggested substitutions to Chart 1 in Appendix A.

Discuss other activities involving the upper extremities. Make a list of those that are similar and those that are different. For example, compare salad preparation at a countertop to brushing one's teeth at the bathroom sink.

REFERENCES

1.   Atkeson CG. Learning arm kinematics and dynamics. *Annu Rev Neurosci.* 1989;12:157-183.

2.   Blakely RL, Palmer ML. Analysis of rotation accompanying shoulder flexion. *Phys Ther.* 1984;64:1214-1216.

3. Bagg SD, Forrest WJ. A biomechanical analysis of scapular rotation during arm abduction in the scapular plane. *Am J Phys Med Rehabil.* 1988;67:238-245.

4. Broome HL, Basmajian JV. The function of the teres major muscle: an electromyographic study. *Anat Rec.* 1970;170:309-310.

5. Dvir Z, Berme N. The shoulder complex in elevation of the arm: a mechanism approach. *J Biomech.* 1978;11:219-225.

6. Freedman L, Munro RR. Abduction of the arm in scapular plane: scapular and glenohumeral movements. *J Bone Joint Surg Am.* 1966;48:1503-1510.

7. Kronberg M, Nemeth G, Brostrom L. Muscle activity and coordination in the normal shoulder. *Clin Orthop.* 1990;257:76-85.

8. Saha AK. Dynamic stability of the glenohumeral joint. *Acta Orthop Scand.* 1971;42:491-505.

9. Walmsley RP, Szybbo C. A comparative study of the torque generated by the shoulder internal and external rotator muscles in different positions and at varying speeds. *J Orthop Sports Phys Ther.* 1987;9:217-222.

10. Basmajian JV, Latif A. Integrated actions and functions of the chief flexors of the elbow: a detailed electromyographic analysis. *J Bone Joint Surg Am.* 1957;39:1106-1118.

11. Ishizuki M. Functional anatomy of the elbow joint and three-dimensional quantitative analysis of the elbow joint. *Journal of the Japanese Orthopedic Association.* 1979;53:986-989.

12. Morrey BF, Askew LJ, An KN, Chao EY. A biomechanical study of normal and functional elbow motion. *J Bone Joint Surg Am.* 1981;63:872-877.

13. Ray RD, Johnson RJ, Jameson RM. Rotation of the forearm: an experimental study of pronation and supination. *J Bone Joint Surg Am.* 1951;33:993-996.

14. Erdman AG, Mayfield JK, Dorman F, Wallrich M, Dahlof W. Kinematic and kinetic analysis of the human wrist by stereoscopic instrumentation. *J Biomech Eng.* 1979;101:124-133.

15. Wadsworth CT. Clinical anatomy and mechanics of the wrist and hand. *J Orthop Sports Phys Ther.* 1983;4:206-216.

16. An KN, Chao EY, Cooney WP, Linscheid RI. Normative model of human hand for biomechanical analysis. *J Biomech.* 1979;12:775-788.

17. Buchholz B, Armstrong TJ. A kinematic model of the human hand to evaluate its prehensile abilities. *J Biomech.* 1992;25:149-162.

18. Chao EY, Opgrande JD, Axmear FE. Three-dimensional force analysis of finger joints in selected isometric hand functions. *J Biomech.* 1976;9:387-396.

19. Landsmeer JMF. Power grip and precision handling. *Ann Rheum Dis.* 1962;21:164-170.

20. Long C, Conrad PW, Hall EA, Furler SL. Intrinsic-extrinsic muscle control of the hand in power grip and precision handling: an electromyographic study. *J Bone Joint Surg Br.* 1970;52:853-867.

21. Bechtol C. Biomechanics of the shoulder. *Clin Orthop*. 1980;146:37-41.
22. Culham E, Peat M. Functional anatomy of the shoulder complex. *J Orthop Sports Phys Ther*. 1993;18:342-350.
23. Gerdle B, Eriksson NE, Hagberg C. Changes in the surface electromyogram during increasing isometric shoulder forward flexion. *Eur J Appl Physiol*. 1988;57:404-408.
24. Jarp Y. Activation of the rotator cuff in generating isometric shoulder rotation torque. *Am J Sports Med*. 1996;24:477-485.
25. Van Woensel W, Arwert H. Effects of external load and abduction angle on EMG level of shoulder muscles during isometric action. *Electromyogr Clin Neurophysiol*. 1993;33:185-191.

SUGGESTED READINGS

An KN, Hui FC, Morrey BF, Linscheid RI, Chao EY. Muscles across the elbow joint: a biomechanical analysis. *J Biomech*. 1981;14:659-669.

Andersson GBJ, Ortengren R, Schultz A. Analysis and measurement of the loads on the lumbar spine during work at a table. *J Biomech*. 1979;17:513-520.

Ayoub MM, LoPresti P. The determination of an optimum size cylindrical handle by use of electromyography. *Ergonomics*. 1971;4:503-518.

Basset RW, Browne AO, Morrey BF, An KN. Glenohumeral muscle force and moment mechanics in a position of shoulder instability. *J Biomech*. 1990;23:405-412.

DeLuca CJ, Forrest WJ. Force analysis of individual muscles acting simultaneously on the shoulder joint during isometric abduction. *J Biomech*. 1973;6:385-393.

Deutsch H, Kilani H, Moustafa E, Hamilton N, Herbert JP. Effect of head-neck position on elbow flexor muscle torque production. *Phys Ther*. 1987;67:517-521.

Hagberg M. Electromyographic signs of shoulder muscular fatigue in two elevated arm positions. *Am J Phys Med Rehabil*. 1981;60:111-121.

Herberts P, Kadefors R, Broman H. Arm positioning in manual tasks—an electromyographic study of localized muscle fatigue. *Ergonomics*. 1980;23:655-665.

Howell SM, Galinat BJ, Renzi AJ. Normal and abnormal mechanics of the glenohumeral joint in the horizontal plane. *J Bone Joint Surg Am*. 1988;70:227-232.

Hsia PT, Drury CG. A simple method of evaluating handle design. *Appl Ergonomics*. 1986;17:209-213.

Jones LA. The assessment of hand function: a critical review of techniques. *J Hand Surg Am*. 1989;14:221-228.

Kauer JMG. Functional anatomy of the wrist. *Clin Orthop*. 1980;149:9-20.

Perry T. Normal upper extremity kinesiology. *Phys Ther*. 1978;58:165-178.

Stroyan M, Wilk KE. The functional anatomy of the elbow complex. *J Orthop Sports Phys Ther.* 1993;17:279-288.

Taylor CL, Schwarz RJ. The anatomy and mechanics of the human hand. *Artificial Limbs.* 1955;2:22-34.

Volz RG, Lieb M, Benjamin J. Biomechanics of the wrist. *Clin Orthop.* 1980;149:112-117.

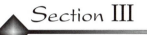

Section III

Lower Extremity
Analyses

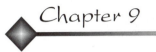

Chapter 9

Donning a Knee-Length Sock

Introduction and Set-Up

People don their socks in many different ways. For instance, some people sit in a chair and bring the foot toward the upper extremities, while others bring the upper extremities toward the foot. Others stand, put one foot on a chair or bed, and bring the upper extremities toward it. The analysis of this activity was limited to the left lower extremity, with the subject seated to perform the task. The sock being used was a knee-length sock.

Preparing to Don the Sock

The activity began with the subject seated, with the hip and knee joints flexed to 90 degrees, the hip midway between internal and external rotation, the ankle joint in neutral, and the feet resting flat on the floor with the metatarsal (MTT) joints in neutral (Figure 9-1). From this position, the subject simultaneously abducted the hip joint 22 degrees and externally rotated the hip 20 degrees; the hip was flexed an additional 17 degrees through this movement.[1-2] Through this motion, the lateral aspect of the leg came to rest on the contralateral knee. The knee joint was maintained in its starting position, as was the ankle joint (Figure 9-2).

The primary muscle involved in this motion was the sartorius, acting concentrically. The external rotators, tensor fascia latae, and iliopsoas muscles, acting concentrically, may be involved but are not needed if the sartorius is strong enough to complete the motion, as was the case with this subject.[3-6] The quadriceps femoris and hamstring muscles worked synergistically to isometrically maintain the knee position.[7-10] The tibialis anterior worked isometrically to maintain the ankle position.[11]

Figure 9-1. Starting position: The subject was seated with feet flat on the floor. The sock was held in the left hand. The key landmarks denoted by black dots are: M = lateral epicondyle of femur; N = fibular head; O = anterior midline between two malleoli; P = lateral malleolus; Q = first MTT joint line (dorsal aspect); R = fifth MTT joint line (lateral aspect); and V = greater trochanter of femur.

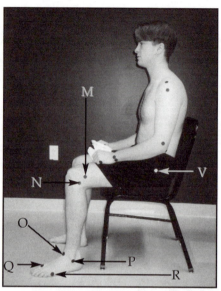

Figure 9-2. Bringing the left lower extremity across the right lower extremity in preparation for donning the sock. The key landmarks denoted by black dots are: O = anterior midline between two malleoli; Q = first MTT joint line (dorsal aspect); R = fifth MTT joint line (lateral aspect); S = midpoint of patella; T = medial malleolus; and U = first MTT joint line (medial aspect).

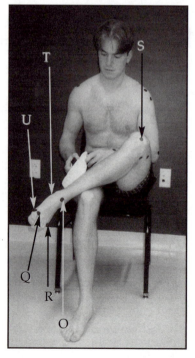

Placing the Sock Over the Foot and Ankle

Next, the subject placed the sock over the foot and ankle. The hip joint flexed an additional 15 degrees and internally rotated back to neutral. The knee and ankle joints remained in their previous positions (Figure 9-3). As the subject continued to pull the sock over the heel (Figure 9-4), the ankle joint was plantarflexed 30 degrees.[12-14]

The iliopsoas and the glutei minimus and medius muscles worked concentrically to position the hip joint.[5,15] The muscles that had been acting on the knee joint continued contracting isometrically to maintain the joint posture. The gastrocnemius-soleus muscle contracted concentrically and drew the ankle joint into plantarflexion.[16] The tibialis posterior and the peronei longus and brevis muscles contracted isometrically to maintain the subtalar joint and foot midway between inversion and eversion.[17-18]

Completing the Donning of the Sock

Once the foot had cleared the opposite knee, the subject began to extend the hip until the posterior thigh touched the chair seat (Figure 9-5). This 32 degrees of extension returned the hip joint to its original starting position of 90 degrees of flexion. The knee joint extended 35 degrees during this time. As the ball of the foot touched the ground, the ankle joint dorsiflexed 10 degrees, allowing the foot to touch the ground (Figure 9-6). All joints distal to the ankle joint were maintained in their previous postures.

The iliopsoas muscle worked eccentrically to control the lowering of the hip joint to its starting position. This eccentric activity resisted the pull of gravity, as well as the weight of the lower extremity, which tends to draw the lower extremity downward.[19] The quadriceps femoris muscle worked concentrically to position the knee joint. The gastrocnemius-soleus muscle also worked eccentrically to allow the ankle joint to dorsiflex.[16-17] All joints distal to the ankle joint were acted upon by isometric muscular contractions to maintain their positions.

Figure 9-3. Placing the sock over the foot: The subject flexed and internally rotated the hip joint. The key landmarks denoted by black dots are: M = lateral epicondyle of femur; N = fibular head; O = anterior midline between two malleoli; and S = midpoint of patella.

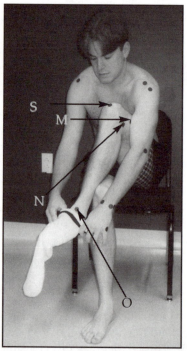

Figure 9-4. Placing the sock over the heel: The subject plantarflexed the ankle joint. The key landmarks denoted by black dots are: M = lateral epicondyle of femur; N = fibular head; and V = greater trochanter of femur.

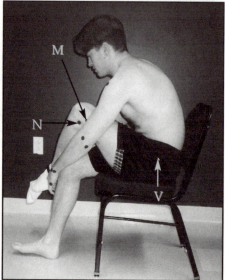

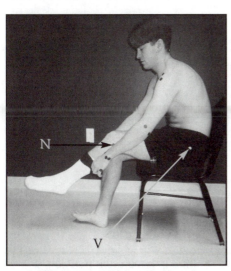

Figure 9-5. Completing the donning of the sock: The subject extended the hip joint, returning the hip to its starting position. The key landmarks denoted by black dots are: N = fibular head and V = greater trochanter of femur.

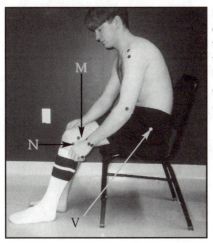

Figure 9-6. Completing the donning of the sock: The foot was returned to the floor as the ankle joint was dorsiflexed. The key landmarks denoted by black dots are: M = lateral epicondyle of femur; N = fibular head; and V = greater trochanter of femur.

Summary

Key Anatomical Landmarks for Knee-Length Sock Analysis

Hip Complex:	Greater trochanter of femur
Knee Complex:	Lateral epicondyle of femur Medial epicondyle of femur Tibial tuberosity Fibular head
Ankle and Foot Complex	Lateral malleolus Medial malleolus Anterior midline between two malleoli First MTT joint line (dorsal aspect) Fifth MTT joint line (lateral aspect)

Major Phases for Knee-Length Sock Analysis

Starting Position
- Position of subject

Placing the Sock Over the Foot and Ankle

Completing the Donning of the Sock

Lower Extremity Joint Motions and Muscular Activity: Donning a Knee-Length Sock

Introduction and Set-Up
- Flexion of hip and knee joints, with ankle joint in neutral.

Preparing to Don the Sock
- Primarily flexion, abduction, and external rotation of hip via concentric muscular contractions.

Placing the Sock Over the Foot and Ankle
- Flexion and internal rotation of hip joint.

• Plantarflexion of ankle joint via concentric muscular contractions.

Completing the Donning of the Sock

• Extension of hip and knee joints via eccentric and concentric muscular activity

• Dorsiflexion of ankle joint via eccentric muscular activity.

CLINICAL APPLICATION AND DISCUSSION QUESTIONS

This analysis was based on a specific technique of donning a knee-length sock. Obviously, the biomechanics would change depending on the technique used. Compare this analysis to keeping the foot on the floor and bringing the upper extremities and the torso toward the lower extremities.

Describe the activity of the upper extremities in donning a knee-length sock. Compare this analysis to that presented in Chapter 6, in which an ankle-length sock was donned. How would the motions of the lower extremities change if an ankle-length sock was applied?

What types of assistive devices could be used if the subject could not flex forward at the hip, as in a patient who recently underwent a total hip replacement? What other types of rehabilitation clients might require assistive devices to dress their lower extremities?

What other activities are comparable to this activity? What are the commonalties? What are the differences?

Generate a list of muscle substitutions for the muscles cited in this chapter's analysis. Compare your substitutions to those in Chart 2 in Appendix A.

REFERENCES

1. Ahlbäck SO, Lindahl O. Sagittal mobility of the hip joint. *Acta Orthop Scand.* 1964;34:310-322.

2. Crowninshield RD, Johnston RC, Andrews JR, Brand RA. A biomechanical investigation of the human hip. *J Biomech.* 1978;11:75-85.

3. Wheatly MD, Jahnke WD. Electromyographic study of the superficial thigh and hip muscles in normal individuals. *Arch Phys Med Rehabil.* 1951;32:508-518.

4. Dostal WF, Andrews JG. A three-dimensional biomechanical model of hip musculature. *J Biomech.* 1981;14:803-812.

5. Haley ET. Range of hip rotation and torque of hip rotator muscle groups. *Am J Phys Med Rehabil.* 1953;32:261-270.

6. Pare EB, Stern JT, Schwartz JM. Functional differentiation within the tensor fasciae latae. *J Bone Joint Surg Am.* 1981;63:1457-1471.

7. Duarte-Cintra AI, Furlani J. Electromyographic study of quadriceps femoris in man. *Electromyogr Clin Neurophysiol.* 1981;21:539-554.

8. Laubenthal KN, Smidt GL, Kettelkamp DB. A quantitative analysis of knee motion during activities of daily living. *Phys Ther.* 1972;52:34-42.

9. Leib FJ, Perry J. Quadriceps function: an electromyographic study under isometric conditions. *J Bone Joint Surg Am.* 1971;53:749-758.

10. Lunnen JD, Yack J, LeVeau BF. Relationship between muscle length, muscle activity, and torque of the hamstring muscles. *Phys Ther.* 1981;61:190-195.

11. Donatelli R. Normal biomechanics of the foot and ankle. *J Orthop Sports Phys Ther.* 1985;7:91-95.

12. Dul J, Johnson GE. A kinematic model of the human ankle. *J Biomech Eng.* 1985;107:137-142.

13. Lundberg A, Goldie I, Kalin B, Selvik G. Kinematics of the ankle/foot complex. 1. Plantarflexion and dorsiflexion. *Foot Ankle Int.* 1989;9:194-200.

14. Sammarco GJ, Burstein AH, Frankel VH. Biomechanics of the ankle: a kinematic study. *Orthop Clin North Am.* 1973;4:75-96.

15. Soderberg GL, Dostal WF. Electromyographic study of three parts of the gluteus medius muscle during functional activities. *Phys Ther.* 1978;58:691-696.

16. Furlani J, Vitti M, Costacurta L. Electromyographic behavior of the gastrocnemius muscle. *Electromyogr Clin Neurophysiol.* 1978;18:29-34.

17. Ambagtsheer JBT. The function of the muscles of the lower leg in relation to movements of the tarsus. *Acta Orthop Scand.* 1978;172(suppl):1-196.

18. Manter JT. Movements of the subtalar and transverse tarsal joints. *Anat Rec.* 1941;80:397-410.

19. Radin EL. Biomechanics of the human hip. *Clin Orthop.* 1980;152:28-34.

SUGGESTED READINGS

Apkarian J, Naumann S, Cairns B. A three-dimensional kinematic and dynamic model of the lower limb. *J Biomech.* 1989;22:143-155.

Brand RA, Crowninshield RD, Johnston RC, Pedersen DR. Forces on the femoral head during activities of daily living. *Iowa Orthop J.* 1982;2:43-49.

Chesworth B. Age and passive ankle stiffness in healthy women. *Phys Ther.* 1989;69:217-224.

Clark JM, Jaynor DR. Anatomy of the abductor muscles of the hips as studied by computer tomography. *J Bone Joint Surg Am.* 1987;69:1021-1031.

Croft P, Cooper C, Wickham C, Coggon D. Osteoarthritis of the hip and occupational activity. *Scand J Work Environ Health.* 1992;18:59-63.

DiStefano V. Anatomy and biomechanics of the ankle and foot. *Athletic Training.* 1981;16:43-47.

Henbusch L. Lightweight inexpensive dressing hook. *Phys Ther.* 1974;54:1202.

Hicks JH. The mechanics of the foot. I. The joints. *J Anat.* 1954;87:345-357.

Johnston RC. Mechanical considerations of the hip joint. *Arch Surg.* 1973;107:411-417.

Lentell GL, Katzman LL, Walters MR. The relationship between muscle function and ankle stability. *J Orthop Sports Phys Ther.* 1990;11:605-611.

Lundberg A, Goldie I, Kalin B, Selvik G. Kinematics of the ankle/foot complex. 2. Pronation and supination. *Foot Ankle Int.* 1989;9:248-253.

Lundberg A, Goldie I, Kalin B, Selvik G. Kinematics of the ankle/foot complex. 3. Influence of leg rotation. *Foot Ankle Int.* 1989;9:304-309.

Lykouretzos J. A folding dressing stick. *Am J Occup Ther.* 1989;44:77.

McLeod WD, Hunter S. Biomechanical analysis of the knee. Primary functions as elucidated by anatomy. *Phys Ther.* 1980;60:1561-1564.

O'Connell AL. Electromyographic study of certain leg muscles during movements of the free foot and during standing. *Am J Phys Med Rehabil.* 1958;37:289-301.

Procter P, Paul JP. Ankle joint biomechanics. *J Biomech.* 1982;15:627-634.

Rydell N. Biomechanics of the hip joint. *Clin Orthop.* 1973;92:6-15.

Reilly DT, Martens M. Experimental analysis of the quadriceps muscle force and patellofemoral joint reaction force for various activities. *Acta Orthop Scand.* 1972;43:126-137.

Rodgers MM. Dynamic foot biomechanics. *J Orthop Sports Phys Ther.* 1995;21:306-316.

Seeger MS, Fisher LA. Adaptive equipment used in the rehabilitation of hip arthroplasty patients. *Am J Occup Ther.* 1982;36:503-508.

Subotnick SI. Biomechanics of the subtalar and midtarsal joints. *J Am Podiatr Med Assoc.* 1975;65:756-764.

Van Kuyk-Minis MAH. Assistive devices: integral to the daily lives of human beings. *Clin Rheum.* 1998;17:3-5.

Wynarsky GT, Greenwald AS. Mathematical model of the human ankle joint. *J Biomech.* 1983;16:241-252.

Chapter 10

Donning a Pair of Pants

INTRODUCTION AND SET-UP

As with any ADL, there are multiple ways in which a pair of pants are donned. Some individuals sit down, pull the pants up to their distal thighs, and then stand to complete the task. Others stand for the entire task. The fit of the pants (tight versus loose), the top opening of the pants (pull-on versus zipper-opening), and the type of material (silk versus corduroy) affect the technique for putting on a pair of pants.

This particular analysis focused on a subject who sits and then stands to put on his pants. The analysis was confined to the motions of the lower extremities. The pants being donned were long-legged, relatively loose-fitting, denim jeans with a front zipper. The analysis started with the subject seated on the edge of a bed. The hip and knee joints were flexed to 90 degrees, with the feet flat on the floor, midway between supination and pronation, and the ankles in neutral. The hips joints were abducted 15 degrees. The subject's upper extremities were flexed, abducted, and internally rotated at the shoulder joints. The elbows were extended, and the forearms were fully pronated. The wrist joints were extended 75 degrees, and the digits were flexed at all joints. The pants were lying on the bed to the subject's left. The upper part of the pants was on the bed, and the lower part was hanging over the side of the bed (Figure 10-1).

REACHING FOR THE PANTS

The subject reached with the left hand to pick up the pants. In doing so, the head and trunk were rotated to the left (Figure 10-2). The lower extremities remained in their starting position. The pants were brought in front of the subject to be grasped by both hands in preparation for donning them.

Figure 10-1. Starting position: The subject was seated with the pants lying to the subject's left. The key landmarks denoted by black dots are: S = midpoint of patella and T = medial malleoli.

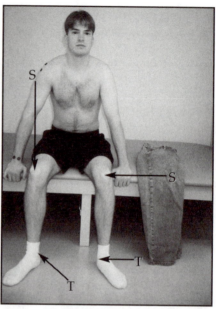

Figure 10-2. Reaching for the pants: The subject rotated the head and trunk to the left while grasping the pants with his left hand. The key landmarks denoted by black dots are: S = midpoint of patella and T = medial malleoli.

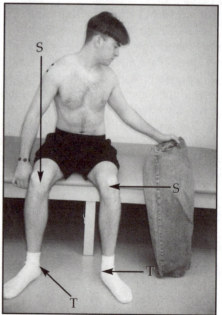

The postural trunk muscles maintained the torso in its upright starting position. The left iliopsoas muscles worked isometrically to assist in maintaining the trunk posture.[1-3] The hamstring muscles worked isometrically to maintain the knee joint position.[4-5] The anterior and posterior tibialis muscles worked isometrically to keep the ankle and foot joints in position.[6-7] The activity of these muscles was important in maintaining upright sitting posture, as the subject's center of gravity was disturbed when he reached backward and to the left to pick up the pants.

DRESSING THE LEFT LOWER EXTREMITY

The subject dressed the left lower extremity first (Figure 10-3). The subject forward flexed the trunk and minimally rotated to the left, while flexing, adducting, and internally rotating the left hip joint. The left hip was flexed 45 degrees, adducted 10 degrees, and internally rotated 5 degrees to bring the foot up toward the hands. The knee joint was flexed an additional 10 degrees.[8]

The ankle joint was dorsiflexed 5 degrees toward the end of this maneuver to position the foot so that the pants could be slipped over the foot. The foot was also inverted 5 degrees.[9-11]

Once the pants were slipped over the foot, the subject began to pull the pants upward over the lower extremity (Figure 10-4). At the same time, the subject lowered the lower extremity to its starting position. During this time, the subject externally rotated and abducted the hip back to its starting position. This placement facilitated dressing of the opposite lower extremity.

As the subject dressed the left lower extremity, the previously cited muscles reversed their activity to eccentric contractions to return the foot to the floor. The right lower extremity muscles then began their work.

DRESSING THE RIGHT LOWER EXTREMITY

The subject repeated the trunk flexion and minimal rotation to the left, while flexing, adducting, and internally rotating the right hip. The right hip joint was flexed an additional 10 degrees, adducted 15 degrees, and internally rotated 10 degrees, which brought the right foot up toward the hands (Figure 10-5). The knee joint flexed 10 degrees. Toward the end of this maneuver, the subject dorsiflexed and inverted the foot to position it for dressing. The ankle joint was dorsiflexed 5 to 10 degrees, and the subtalar joint was inverted 5 degrees.

Figure 10-3. Dressing the left lower extremity: The subject flexed, adducted, and internally rotated the left hip joint, while flexing the knee joint, dorsiflexing the ankle joint, and inverting the foot. The key landmarks denoted by black dots are: S = midpoint of patella and T = medial malleoli.

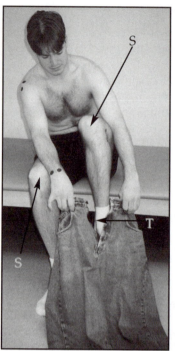

Figure 10-4. Dressing the left lower extremity: The subject flexed, adducted, and internally rotated the left hip joint. The key landmarks denoted by black dots are: M = lateral epicondyle of femur; N = fibular head; and V = greater trochanter of femur.

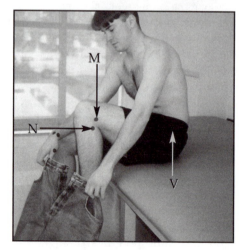

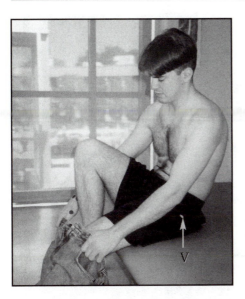

Figure 10-5. Dressing the right lower extremity: The subject flexed, adducted, and internally rotated the right hip joint. The key landmark denoted by the black mark is V = greater trochanter of femur.

The subject slipped the pants over the right foot and pulled the pants upward. At the same time, the subject lowered the right lower extremity to the floor (Figure 10-6). As with the left side, the right lower extremity was returned to its starting position, including a neutral position for internal and external rotation. The subject returned the trunk to the upright starting position. The muscles involved in dressing the right lower extremity were the mirror images of the left lower extremity muscles. Their activity was the same as that cited for the left lower extremity.

COMPLETION OF DONNING THE PANTS

The subject was now ready to complete the donning of the pants by standing up. While keeping the grasp on the pants, the subject flexed forward at the waist to prepare for weight transfer to the lower extremity. Simultaneously, the subject extended the hip and knee joints, which forced the ankles into dorsiflexion.[4] Initially, the hip joints flexed 10 degrees (Figure 10-7) and then began to move toward full extension. The knee joints initially flexed an additional 5 degrees before moving to full extension.[4] The ankle joints dorsiflexed 5 degrees and then moved toward plantarflexion, coming to rest in the neutral position.[12-13] As this movement was occurring, the subject's trunk returned to the upright position, while the subject pulled the pants up over the thighs and hips and completed the donning of the pants (Figures 10-8).

Figure 10-6. Dressing the right lower extremity: As the subject pulled the pants upward, the right lower extremity was lowered to the floor. The key landmark denoted by the black dot is V = greater trochanter of femur.

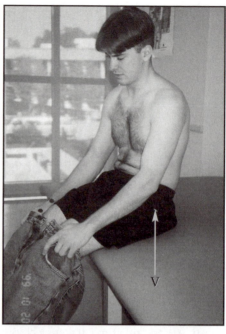

Figure 10-7. Completion of donning the pants: The subject dorsiflexed the hip and knee joints to initiate weight transfer to the lower extremities. The key landmarks denoted by black dots are: R = fifth MTT joint line (lateral aspect) and V = greater trochanter of femur.

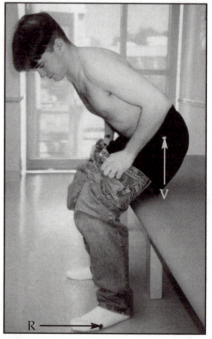

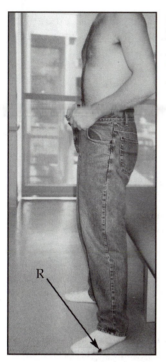

Figure 10-8. Completion of donning the pants: The pants were in their final position to be zipped. The key landmark denoted by the black dot is R = fifth MTT joint line (lateral aspect).

In preparation for standing, the iliopsoas muscle (working concentrically) and the gluteus maximus muscle (working eccentrically) moved the hip joints into the initial flexion component. The gluteus maximus muscle then reversed its activity to concentric contractions, which moved the hip joint into its extended position.[14]

The motion at the knee and ankle joints (the initial increased flexion) was passive in nature due to the forward progression of the trunk, while the foot was held against the floor. Once the knees moved toward extension, the quadriceps femoris muscle worked concentrically.[15-16] At the ankle joint, the gastrocnemius-soleus muscle worked concentrically as the full upright standing posture was reached. The tibialis anterior worked synergistically with the gastrocnemius-soleus muscle to achieve this final position. Eccentric contractions of the tibialis anterior were needed to stabilize the ankle as the subject pulled the pants over the hips and pelvis.[6,17] There was also an interplay between the invertors and evertors of the subtalar joint to stabilize the foot against the floor.[11] While the tibialis posterior worked concentrically, the peronei longus and brevis muscles worked eccentrically. This then switched so that both muscles worked in reverse. This allowed a small amount of inversion and eversion to stabilize the subject's upright posture while the pants were finally positioned on the subject.

SUMMARY

Key Anatomical Landmarks for Pants Analysis

Hip Complex:	Greater trochanter of femur
Knee Complex:	Lateral epicondyle of femur Medial epicondyle of femur Tibial tuberosity Fibular head Midpoint of patella
Ankle and Foot Complex:	Lateral malleolus Medial malleolus Anterior midline between two malleoli First MTT joint line (dorsal aspect) First MTT joint line (medial aspect) Fifth MTT joint line (lateral aspect)

Major Phases for Pants Analysis

Starting Position
- Position of subject
- Position of pants
- Type of pants

Reaching for the Pants

Dressing the Left Lower Extremity

Dressing the Right Lower Extremity

Completion of Donning the Pants

Lower Extremity Joint Motion and Muscular Activity: Donning a Pair of Pants

Introduction and Set-Up
• Flexion and abduction of hip joint.

• Knee joint in flexion and ankle joints in neutral.

Reaching for the Pants
• All joints are maintaining their positions via isometric muscular activity.

Dressing the Left Lower Extremity
• Primarily flexion of all joints.

• Extension of hip joint via concentric muscular activity.

Dressing the Right Lower Extremity
• Primarily flexion of all joints.

• Extension of hip joint via concentric muscular activity.

Completion of Donning the Pants
• Primarily flexion of all joints.

• Extension of hip and knee joints via concentric muscular activity.

CLINICAL APPLICATION AND DISCUSSION QUESTIONS

This analysis was based on a sit-and-stand technique. The amount of motion produced at the hip, knee, and ankle joints will vary with different techniques, as will the muscular activity. Proprioceptive and balance abilities of an individual will enter into the choice of technique to complete this task.

Describe the performance of this activity in the standing position. This will require momentarily balancing on one lower extremity while dressing the opposite lower extremity. Consider the trunk and upper extremity motions that will be needed to don the pants in this position.

What is the impact of balance problems on completing this activity as presented in this chapter and on completing this activity in the standing position?

Compare this activity to donning a tight-fitting pair of pants. How does the activity change?

Compare this activity to donning a pair of socks or pantyhose. What are the similarities? What are the differences?

What types of assistive devices might be appropriate for those individuals who have difficulty completing this activity due to involvement of the lower or upper extremities? What other ways of performing this activity would be appropriate for those individuals with sitting and/or standing balance impairments?

Finally, list muscle substitutions for the prime movers of these analyses. Compare your choices to those muscles listed in Chart 2 in Appendix A.

REFERENCES

1. Dostal WF, Andrews JG. A three-dimensional biomechanical model of hip musculature. *J Biomech.* 1981;14:803-812.

2. Radin EL. Biomechanics of the human hip. *Clin Orthop.* 1980;152:28-34.

3. Wheatly MD, Jahnke WD. Electromyographic study of the superficial thigh and hip muscles in normal individuals. *Arch Phys Med Rehabil.* 1951;32:508-518.

4. Laubenthal KN, Smidt GL, Kettelkamp DB. A quantitative analysis of knee motion during activities of daily living. *Phys Ther.* 1972;52:34-42.

5. Lunnen JD, Yack J, LeVeau BF. Relationship between muscle length, muscle activity, and torque of the hamstring muscles. *Phys Ther.* 1981;61:190-195.

6. Ambagtsheer JBT. The function of the muscles of the lower leg in relation to movements of the tarsus. *Acta Orthop Scand.* 1978;172(suppl):1-19.

7. Procter P, Paul JP. Ankle joint biomechanics. *J Biomech.* 1982;15:627-634.

8. Chari VR, Kirby RL. Lower-limb influence on sitting balance while reaching forward. *Arch Phys Med Rehabil.* 1986;67:730-733.

9. Donatelli R. Normal biomechanics of the foot and ankle. *J Orthop Sports Phys Ther.* 1985;7:91-95.

10. Lundberg A, Goldie I, Kalin B, Selvik G. Kinematics of the ankle/foot complex. 2. Pronation and supination. *Foot Ankle Int.* 1989;9:248-253.

11. Subotnick SI. Biomechanics of the subtalar and midtarsal joints. *J Am Podiatr Med Assoc.* 1975;65:756-764.

12. Lundberg A, Goldie I, Kalin B, Selvik G. Kinematics of the ankle/foot complex. 1. Plantarflexion and dorsiflexion. *Foot Ankle Int.* 1989;9:194-200.

13. Lundberg A, Goldie I, Kalin B, Selvik G. Kinematics of the ankle/foot complex. 3. Influence of leg rotation. *Foot Ankle Int*. 1989;9:304-309.

14. Yamashita N. EMG activities in mono- and bi-articular thigh muscles in combined hip and knee extension. *Eur J Appl Physiol*. 1988;58:274-277.

15. Duarte-Cintra AI, Furlani J. Electromyographic study of quadriceps femoris in man. *Electromyogr Clin Neurophysiol*. 1981;21:539-554.

16. Reilly DT, Martens M. Experimental analysis of the quadriceps muscle force and patellofemoral joint reaction force for various activities. *Acta Orthop Scand*. 1972;43:126-137.

17. Lentell GL, Katzman LL, Walters MR. The relationship between muscle function and ankle stability. *J Orthop Sports Phys Ther*. 1990;11:605-611.

SUGGESTED READINGS

Blackburn TA, Craig E. Knee anatomy: a brief review. *Phys Ther*. 1980;60:1556-1560.

Brand RA, Crowninshield RD, Johnston RC, Pedersen DR. Forces on the femoral head during activities of daily living. *Iowa Orthop J*. 1982;2:43-49.

Johnston RC. Mechanical considerations of the hip joint. *Arch Surg*. 1973;107:411-417.

Nissan M. Review of some basic assumptions in knee biomechanics. *J Biomech*. 1980;13:375-381.

Sammarco GJ, Burstein AH, Frankel VH. Biomechanics of the ankle: a kinematic study. *Orthop Clin North Am*. 1973;4:75-96.

Shepard E. Tarsal movements. *J Bone Joint Surg Br*. 1951;33:258-263.

Van Kuyk-Minis MAH. Assistive devices: integral to the daily lives of human beings. *Clin Rheum*. 1998;17:3-5.

Chapter 11

Mounting and Pedaling a Bicycle

INTRODUCTION AND SET-UP

Young and old alike enjoy bicycling. In this muscular analysis, bicycling was broken down into two main phases: mounting the bicycle and pedaling the bicycle. The last main phase was further subdivided into four components. Each component was made up of one quarter of a complete pedal cycle, with the pedal cycle being designated similar to the face of the clock, using a counter-clockwise direction for the left lower extremity and a clockwise direction for the right lower extremity. The four components included the 12 o'clock, 9 o'clock, 6 o'clock, and 3 o'clock positions. The 3 o'clock range of motion (ROM) measurement was taken at 270 degrees; the 6 o'clock ROM at 180 degrees; the 9 o'clock ROM at 90 degrees; and the 12 o'clock position at 360 or 0 degrees. The extremity had completed a pedal cycle when it had gone from a point equivalent to 12 o'clock, through a ROM, and returned to that original 12 o'clock position. For the purposes of this analysis, the activity was limited to the pedaling cycle of the left lower extremity.

A standard stationary bicycle was used for this analysis in order to obtain ROM measurements without the need of assistants to stabilize a regular bicycle. The saddle seat height of the bicycle was set at 30 inches from the floor. This measurement put the seat height at the height of the subject's femoral greater trochanter (Figure 11-1).

MOUNTING THE BICYCLE

For the first main phase (mounting the bicycle), the subject started in a static position, with the hip, knee, and ankle joints in their neutral position and no appreciable motion occurring. As the subject mounted

Figure 11-1. Starting position: The subject stood to the left of the bicycle. The saddle seat was set at a height equivalent to the subject's femoral greater trochanter. The key landmarks denoted by black dots are: M = lateral epicondyle of femur; N = fibular head; O = anterior midline between two malleoli; P = lateral malleolus; Q = first MTT joint line (dorsal aspect); R = fifth MTT joint line (lateral aspect); and V = greater trochanter of femur.

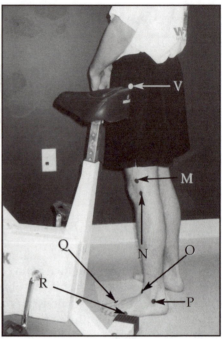

the bicycle, he went through a series of rapid, successive movements while maintaining upright balance. The right pelvis was laterally tilted downward, while the left hip was abducted and flexed to bring the extremity up and over the saddle seat.[1-2] Simultaneously, the left knee joint was flexed, while the ankle joint was held in a neutral position (Figure 11-2).

As the mounting proceeded, the right pelvis laterally tilted 4 to 5 degrees. The left hip joint abducted 35 degrees, flexed 100 degrees, and internally rotated 5 degrees, while the knee joint flexed to approximately 90 degrees.[3-6] The left ankle joint was held in a neutral position to help clear the toes over the bike (Figure 11-3). The left hip joint then moved into extension and returned to approximately 12 degrees of flexion. The left hip joint remained abducted approximately 5 to 10 degrees. The left knee joint moved to 20 degrees of flexion to place the foot on the pedal. The left ankle joint remained in the neutral position (Figure 11-4).

Now that the left lower extremity had been positioned, the right lower extremity was moved to place the right foot on its pedal. Weight was shifted to the left side to unload the right lower extremity, which had been bearing the body weight during the first part of the mounting phase.[7]

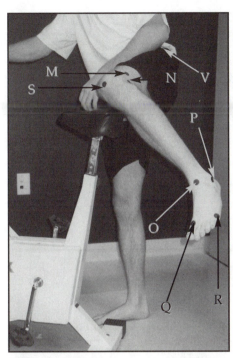

Figure 11-2. Mounting the bicycle: The subject began to bring the left lower extremity over the seat by abducting and flexing the hip joint while simultaneously flexing the knee joint. The key landmarks denoted by black dots are: M = lateral epicondyle of femur; N = fibular head; O = anterior midline between two malleoli; P = lateral malleolus; Q = first MTT joint line (dorsal aspect); R = fifth MTT joint line (lateral aspect); S = midpoint of patella; and V = greater trochanter of femur.

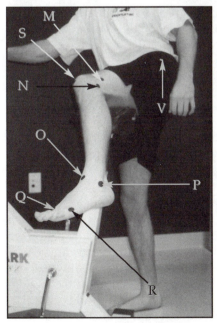

Figure 11-3. Mounting the bicycle: The subject had cleared the seat and was ready to start the transfer of weight to the left lower extremity. The key landmarks denoted by black dots are: M = lateral epicondyle of femur; N = fibular head; O = anterior midline between two malleoli; P = lateral malleolus; Q = first MTT joint line (dorsal aspect); R = fifth MTT joint line (lateral aspect); S = midpoint of patella; and V = greater trochanter of femur.

Figure 11-4. Mounting the bicycle: The subject has seated himself on the saddle seat and transferred weight to the left lower extremity. The key landmarks denoted by black dots are: M = lateral epicondyle of femur; N = fibular head; O = anterior midline between two malleoli; P = lateral malleolus; Q = first MTT joint line (dorsal aspect); R = fifth MTT joint line (lateral aspect); and V = greater trochanter of femur.

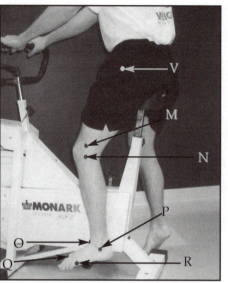

The right ankle joint was plantarflexed 50 degrees, while the left hip joint externally rotated to a neutral position, and the right pelvis returned to a neutral position (Figure 11-5).

The right hip joint was flexed 30 degrees, while the right knee joint was flexed 45 degrees to place the right foot on the pedal. This resulted in the right ankle joint being dorsiflexed 5 to 10 degrees once the right foot was on the pedal (Figure 11-6).

Starting from the bilateral stance phase prior to mounting the bicycle, static stabilizers were active to maintain the body in its upright position.[7-10] This muscle analysis began as the subject started to mount the bicycle. The subject's right lower extremity was the stance leg as the left lower extremity was moved up and over the saddle seat. The left quadratus lumborum and the right gluteus medius, both acting concentrically, controlled the lateral tilting of the pelvis.[10-15] The right gluteus maximus, quadriceps femoris, and gastrocnemius-soleus muscles stabilized the right lower extremity during this mounting phase. This was accomplished by isometric activity of these muscles.

The muscles acting at the left hip and knee joints primarily performed concentrically, while the ankle joint muscles worked eccentrically to control the ankle joint position. The left iliopsoas, gluteus medius, external rotators, quadriceps femoris, and tibialis anterior controlled the motions as the left lower extremity was brought up and over the saddle seat. The hip muscles worked concentrically to flex and abduct the hip joint.

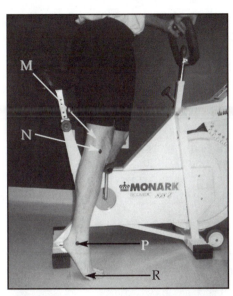

Figure 11-5. Mounting the bicycle: The subject plantarflexed the right ankle joint to shift his weight to the left lower extremity. The key landmarks denoted by black dots are: M = lateral epicondyle of femur; N = fibular head; P = lateral malleolus; and R = fifth MTT joint line (lateral aspect).

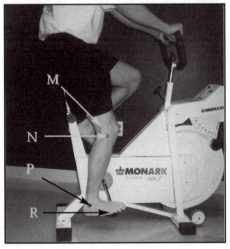

Figure 11-6. Completion of mounting the bicycle: The subject placed the right foot on the pedal. The key landmarks denoted by black dots are: M = lateral epicondyle of femur; N = fibular head; P = lateral malleolus; and R = fifth MTT joint line (lateral aspect).

The external rotators worked eccentrically to control the amount of internal rotation at the hip joint.[16] The knee muscles worked eccentrically to control the amount of knee flexion. The ankle dorsiflexors worked isometrically to maintain the neutral position of the ankle joint. In addition, the peronei longus and brevis worked isometrically to help maintain the position of the subtalar joint during this time.[17-18]

Once over the saddle seat, the left iliopsoas worked eccentrically to lower the hip joint into position as the foot was placed on the pedal. The left gluteus medius worked eccentrically to lessen the amount of abduction of the hip joint. The external rotators worked concentrically to return the hip joint to a neutral position. The left quadriceps femoris continued to work eccentrically to control the motion of the knee as the knee joint proceeded toward a more extended position. The ankle dorsiflexors sustained an isometric contraction to keep the ankle joint positioned. The evertors of the subtalar joint worked eccentrically to allow the foot to be placed evenly on the pedal.

The right gastrocnemius-soleus muscles worked concentrically to push the body upward and shift the weight to the opposite side, so the right foot could be brought into position on its pedal. At the same time, there was a concentric contraction of the right evertors as weight was shifted to the medial border of the right foot during this upward thrust of the body.[19] The left gluteus medius began to contract concentrically to level the pelvis. It then switched to an isometric contraction to maintain this position until the right foot was on its pedal.[11]

The right iliopsoas muscles worked concentrically to flex the hip joint and assist in placing the right foot on its pedal. The right quadriceps femoris muscles worked eccentrically to control the amount of knee flexion needed. The right dorsiflexors and invertors worked concentrically to bring the ankle and subtalar joints into position as the foot was placed on its pedal. The subject was now ready to begin pedaling.

PEDALING THE BICYCLE

The other main phase (pedaling) was described from the perspective of the previously-mentioned clock face. The left lower extremity started with the foot at the 12 o'clock position (Figure 11-7) and pressed forward and downward. From this position, the hip joint started at a flexed position of 88 degrees, the knee joint at 115 degrees of flexion, the ankle joint at neutral, and the MTP joint in neutral.[20-25]

From here, the foot pedaled toward the 9 o'clock position and completed a quarter of the pedal cycle (Figure 11-8). The hip joint was now in 66 degrees of flexion, the knee joint in 75 degrees of flexion, and the ankle joint in 15 degrees of plantarflexion. The MTP joint remained in neutral.

Continuing the pedaling motion, the foot moved toward the 6 o'clock position, completing half of the pedal cycle (Figure 11-9). The hip joint was now flexed 38 degrees, the knee joint flexed 45 degrees, and the ankle joint plantarflexed 10 degrees. The MTP joints remained in neutral.

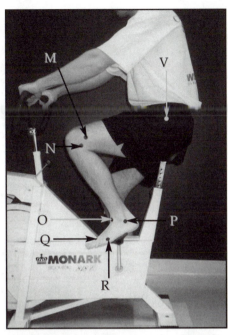

Figure 11-7. Pedaling the bicycle: The left lower extremity started with the foot at the 12 o'clock position. The key landmarks denoted by black dots are: M = lateral epicondyle of femur; N = fibular head; O = anterior midline between two malleolli; P = lateral malleolus; Q = first MTT joint line (dorsal aspect); R = fifth MTT joint line (lateral aspect); and V = greater trochanter of femur.

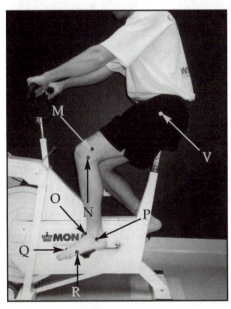

Figure 11-8. Pedaling the bicycle: The foot moved into the 9 o'clock position. The key landmarks denoted by black dots are: M = lateral epicondyle of femur; N = fibular head; O = anterior midline between two malleoli; P = lateral malleolus; Q = first MTT joint line (dorsal aspect); R = fifth MTT joint line (lateral aspect); and V = greater trochanter of femur.

Figure 11-9. Pedaling the bicycle: Half of the pedal cycle was completed, with the foot now at the 6 o'clock position. The key landmarks denoted by black dots are: M = lateral epicondyle of femur; N = fibular head; O = anterior midline between two malleoli; P = lateral malleolus; Q = first MTT joint line (dorsal aspect); R = fifth MTT joint line (lateral aspect); and V = greater trochanter of femur.

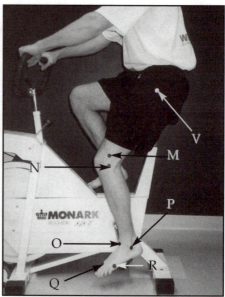

From here, the foot moved toward the 3 o'clock position and completed three-quarters of the pedal cycle (Figure 11-10). The hip joint flexed to 60 degrees, the knee joint flexed to 95 degrees, the ankle joint returned to neutral, and the MTP joints remained in neutral.

Finally, the foot moved toward the 12 o'clock position (Figure 11-11), completed the pedal cycle, and returned to its original starting position. It should also be noted that the subtalar joint inverted and everted throughout the pedaling cycle. There was approximately 4 degrees of motion in either direction.

Pedaling the bicycle was a repetitive motion of bilateral limb motions. Therefore, muscle activity demonstrated in one limb was analogous to that of the opposite limb. However, when one limb was at the 12 o'clock position, the opposite limb was at the 6 o'clock position. The muscle activity described here was limited to the left lower extremity for purposes of this analysis.

It is important to remember that pedaling occurred in a counter-clockwise motion as the subject was observed from his left side. Starting at the 12 o'clock position, the subject moved from 0 to 90 degrees. During this time, the subject moved from a flexed hip and knee posture to an extended hip and knee posture, and then back to a flexed hip and knee posture. During the first part of the pedal cycle, the gluteus maximus acted concentrically by moving the hip joint in an extension component, thereby

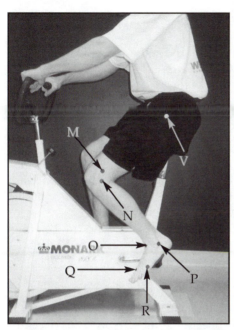

Figure 11-10. Pedaling the bicycle: The foot was at the 3 o'clock position, having completed three-quarters of the pedal cycle. The key landmarks denoted by black dots are: M = lateral epicondyle of femur; N = fibular head; O = anterior midline between two malleoli; P = lateral malleolus; Q = first MTT joint line (dorsal aspect); R = fifth MTT joint line (lateral aspect); and V = greater trochanter of femur.

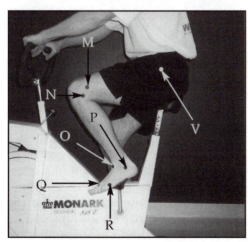

Figure 11-11. Pedaling the bicycle: The pedal cycle was completed with the return of the foot to the 12 o'clock position. The key landmarks denoted by black dots are: M = lateral epicondyle of femur; N = fibular head; O = anterior midline between two malleoli; P = lateral malleolus; Q = first MTT joint line (dorsal aspect); R = fifth MTT joint line (lateral aspect); and V = greater trochanter of femur.

decreasing the amount of initial flexion. The quadriceps femoris muscle acting concentrically, and the hamstrings acting eccentrically, moved the knee toward extension, decreasing the amount of initial flexion of the knee joint. The gastrocnemius-soleus muscle acted concentrically to plantarflex the ankle joint. The peronei longus and brevis muscles acted concentrically to control the movement of the subtalar joint. This entire motion was a downward thrust of the left lower extremity to propel the bicycle forward.[26-29]

In addition, the hamstring and hip adductor muscles worked eccentrically to help control the motion. However, the adductor magnus muscle worked concentrically during the second half of this downward thrust component of the pedal cycle. The tibialis anterior, working eccentrically, also helped to control the motion.

During the second part of the pedal cycle, the pedal was moved from the 9 o'clock position to the 6 o'clock position, or from 90 to 180 degrees. The same muscle activity cited for the first part of the pedal cycle persisted, driving the pedal downward.

As the pedal continued to move from the 6 o'clock position to the 3 o'clock position, or from 180 to 270 degrees, the hip flexors, iliopsoas, sartorius, tensor fasciae latae, and pectineus muscles worked concentrically to produce the hip joint motion. The hamstrings and gracilis muscles worked concentrically to produce knee flexion, assisted by eccentric activity of the quadriceps femoris muscle. The ankle dorsiflexion was produced by a concentric contraction of the tibialis anterior muscle.

To complete the pedal cycle and bring the foot back to the 12 o'clock starting position, the foot moved from 270 to 360 degrees. The hip flexor and the knee flexor muscles continued to act concentrically to produce this motion. The tibialis anterior muscle contracted isometrically to maintain the ankle joint position. The gastrocnemius-soleus muscle worked synergistically with the tibialis anterior muscle to control the ankle joint.

In addition to the above muscles, the hip rotator (medial and lateral), adductor, and abductor muscles were working as stabilizers to keep the left lower extremity in a neutral position. The pelvic elevators worked continuously to maintain the level of the pelvis in a position to foster maximum use of the lower extremities. The same concept applied to the ankle invertors and evertors to stabilize the foot on the pedal. It should also be noted that the adductor magnus muscle would work concentrically as a hip extensor when resistance was added to the pedaling motion, such as can be done with an exercise device like a restorator.[30-31]

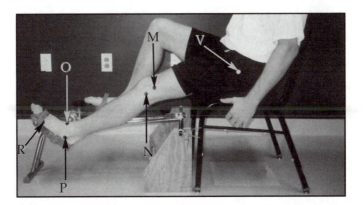

Figure 11-12. Starting position for the restorator: The pedals were set 30 inches from the subject's femoral greater trochanter. The key landmarks denoted by black dots are: M = lateral epicondyle of femur; N = fibular head; O = anterior mid-line between two malleoli; P = lateral malleolus; R = fifth MTT joint line (lateral aspect); and V = greater trochanter of femur.

COMPARISON TO AN ERGOMETER AND A RESTORATOR

The motions and muscle activities for mounting and pedaling an ergometer were the same as those cited for a bicycle. The main difference was in the proprioceptive and balance abilities needed by the individual who was riding a standard bicycle, as there were no external supports to maintain the bicycle in its upright position.

When this analysis was compared to that of pedaling a restorator, a few differences were noted. To set the foot pedals at an appropriate distance, the subject was seated in a chair and asked to extend the left knee. The restorator pedals were set at a distance of 30 inches from the femoral greater trochanter (Figure 11-12), with the subject in this position.

At the starting position of 12 o'clock, or 0 degrees (Figure 11-13), the hip joint was in 95 degrees of flexion, the knee joint in 105 degrees of flexion, and the ankle joint in 5 degrees of plantarflexion. Moving from 0 to 90 degrees (see Figure 11-12), the hip joint moved to 70 degrees of flexion, the knee joint to 10 degrees of flexion, and the ankle joint to 15 degrees of plantarflexion.

Moving from 90 to 180 degrees (Figure 11-14), the hip joint increased its ROM to 86 degrees of flexion; the knee joint increased to 91 degrees of flexion; and the ankle joint returned to a neutral position. Continuing to 270 degrees (Figure 11-15), the hip joint flexed to 88 degrees; the knee

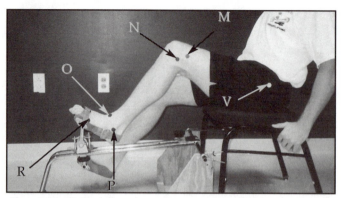

Figure 11-13. Pedaling the restorator: The subject started at the 12 o'clock position. The key landmarks denoted by black dots are: M = lateral epicondyle of femur; N = fibular head; O = anterior midline between two malleolli; P = lateral malleolus; R = fifth MTT joint line (lateral aspect); and V = greater trochanter of femur.

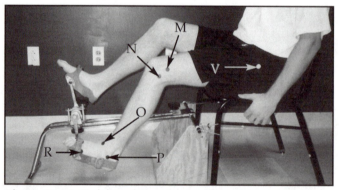

Figure 11-14. Pedaling the restorator: The subject moved from the 9 o'clock to the 6 o'clock position. The key landmarks denoted by black dots are: M = lateral epicondyle of femur; N = fibular head; O = anterior midline between two malleoli; P = lateral malleolus; R = fifth MTT joint line (lateral aspect); and V = greater trochanter of femur.

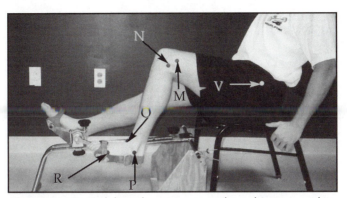

Figure 11-15. Pedaling the restorator: The subject moved to the 3 o'clock position, completing three-quarters of the pedal cycle. The key landmarks denoted by black dots are: M = lateral epicondyle of femur; N = fibular head; O = anterior midline between two malleoli; P = lateral malleolus; R = fifth MTT joint line (lateral aspect); and V = greater trochanter of femur.

joint flexed to 90 degrees; and the ankle joint remained in neutral. During the entire pedal cycle, the MTP and interphalangeal joints were flexed 15, 90, 45, and 10 degrees, respectively. This flexion enabled the subject to maintain his grip on the pedal.

The muscles producing these motions were essentially the same as those listed for the bicycle. In addition, the flexors digitorum longus and brevis, hallucis longus, and digiti minimi muscles worked isometrically to maintain the foot's grasp on the pedal. As with the bicycle, there was synergistic muscular activity to control and stabilize the joints of the lower extremity.

SUMMARY

Key Anatomical Landmarks for Bicycle Analysis

Hip Complex:	Greater trochanter of femur
	Anterior superior iliac spines
	Iliac crests (posterior aspect)
Knee Complex:	Lateral epicondyle of femur
	Midpoint of patella
	Fibular head

Ankle and Foot Complex:	Lateral malleolus
	Anterior midline between two malleoli
	First MTT joint line (dorsal aspect)
	Fifth MTT joint line (lateral aspect)

Major Phases for Bicycle Analysis

Starting Position
- Position of subject

- Type of bicycle

- Position of saddle seat

Mounting the Bicycle
- Left lower extremity

- Right lower extremity

Pedaling the Bicycle
- From 12 o'clock to 9 o'clock position

- From 9 o'clock to 6 o'clock position

- From 6 o'clock to 3 o'clock position

- From 3 o'clock to 12 o'clock position

Lower Extremity Joint Motions and Muscular Activity: Mounting and Pedaling a Bicycle

Introduction and Set-Up
- All joints started in a neutral position.

Mounting the Bicycle
- Primarily downward lateral tilting of right pelvis.

- Flexion of left hip and knee joints followed by extension of left hip and knee joints.

- Combination of concentric and eccentric muscular contractions followed by primarily flexion of right hip, knee, and ankle joints via concentric muscular contractions.

Pedaling the Bicycle

- Primarily moving from flexion to extension to flexion of hip, knee, and ankle joints.

- Primarily concentric muscular contractions.

Comparison to Restorator

- Essentially the same throughout the pedaling cycle.

Major Differences in Pedaling an Ergometer and a Restorator

- Lower extremity is angulated perpendicular to floor with bicycle and ergometer.

- Lower extremity is angulated parallel to floor with restorator.

- Less ROM needed with restorator.

CLINICAL APPLICATION AND DISCUSSION QUESTIONS

As seen from this analysis, the bicycle and ergometer require a greater total excursion for all motions.[20-21,23] However, the end range of hip and knee flexion was greater with the restorator. Adjustments could be made on any of these devices to account for limited range of motion and continued use of any device. The main exception would be in the case of an individual whose lower extremity length exceeded the capacity of the device used.

This analysis focused on the lower extremity motions and muscles. Describe the trunk and upper extremity postures when bicycling. Compare this to the trunk and upper extremity motions when using an ergometer with moving handlebars that are attached to the foot pedals. Then compare this to the trunk and upper extremity postures when using a restorator. What muscles are needed in each of these situations?

Look at the use of toe clips on a bicycle. Will the lower extremity muscular activity change for the individual who uses toe clips? If so, how? In addition, look at the foot position on the pedal. Does the individual pedal with the ball of the foot, the midportion of the foot, or the heel of the foot on the pedal? Does the individual externally or internally rotate the foot on the pedal or keep it aligned in the midposition? Will any of these position changes alter the muscular activity of the lower extremity? How will this muscular analysis change if the subject pedaled the bicycle while standing the entire time? How will this activity change if the bicycle is pedaled through an upper extremity mechanism?

Finally, list muscle substitutions for the prime movers. Compare your list with Chart 2 in Appendix A.

REFERENCES

1. Drerup B, Hierholzer E. Movement of the human pelvis and displacement of related anatomical landmarks on the body surface. *J Biomech.* 1987;20:971-977.

2. Crowninshield RD, Johnston RC, Andrews JR, Brand RA. A biomechanical investigation of the human hip. *J Biomech.* 1978;11:75-85.

3. Blacharski K, Somerset JH. A three-dimensional study of the kinematics of the human knee. *J Biomech.* 1988;8:375-384.

4. Blackburn TA, Craig E. Knee anatomy: a brief review. *Phys Ther.* 1980;60:1556-1560.

5. Smidt GL. Biomechanical analysis of knee flexion and extension. *J Biomech.* 1973;6:79-92.

6. Sammarco GJ, Burstein AH, Frankel VH. Biomechanics of the ankle: a kinematic study. *Orthop Clin North Am.* 1973;4:75-96.

7. Apkarian J, Naumann S, Cairns B. A three-dimensional kinematic and dynamic model of the lower limb. *J Biomech.* 1989;22:143-155.

8. Dostal WF, Andrews JG. A three-dimensional biomechanical model of hip musculature. *J Biomech.* 1981;14:803-821.

9. Fisk R, Wells J. The quadriceps complex in bipedal man. *J Am Osteopath Assoc.* 1980;80:291-294.

10. Lentell GL, Katzman LL, Walters MR. The relationship between muscle function and ankle stability. *J Orthop Sports Phys Ther.* 1990;11:605-611.

11. Soderberg GL, Dostal WF. Electromyographic study of three parts of the gluteus medius muscle during functional activities. *Phys Ther.* 1978;58:691-696.

12. Inman VT. Functional aspects of the abductor muscles of the hip. *J Bone Joint Surg Am.* 1947;29:607-619.

13. Duarte-Cintra AI, Furlani J. Electromyographic study of quadriceps femoris in man. *Electromyogr Clin Neurophysiol.* 1981;21:539-554.

14. Leib FJ, Perry J. Quadriceps function: an electromyographic study under isometric conditions. *J Bone Joint Surg Am.* 1971;53:749-758.

15. Furlani J, Vitti M, Costacurta L. Electromyographic behavior of the gastrocnemius muscle. *Electromyogr Clin Neurophysiol.* 1978;18:29-34.
16. Haley ET. Range of hip rotation and torque of hip rotator muscle groups. *Am J Phys Med Rehabil.* 1953;32:261-270.
17. Subotnick SI. Biomechanics of the subtalar and midtarsal joints. *J Am Podiatr Med Assoc.* 1975;65:756-764.
18. Manter JT. Movements of the subtalar and transverse tarsal joints. *Anat Rec.* 1941;80:397-410.
19. Ambagtsheer JBT. The function of the muscles of the lower leg in relation to movements of the tarsus. *Acta Orthop Scand.* 1978;172(suppl):1-196.
20. Houtz SJ, Fischer FJ. An analysis of muscle action and joint excursion during exercise on a stationary bicycle. *J Bone Joint Surg Am.* 1959;41:123-131.
21. Neptune RR, Hull ML. Accuracy assessment of methods for determining hip movement in seated cycling. *J Biomech.* 1995;28:423-437.
22. Redfield R, Hull ML. On the relation between joint moments and pedaling rates at constant power in cycling. *J Biomech.* 1986;19:317-324.
23. Ericson MO, Nisell R, Nemeth G. Joint motions of the lower limb during ergometer cycling. *J Orthop Sports Phys Ther.* 1988;9:273-278.
24. Ericson MO, Bratt A, Nisell R, Arborelius UP, Ekholm J. Load moments about the hip and knee joints during ergometer cycling. *Scand J Rehabil Med.* 1986;18:165-172.
25. Ericson MO, Bratt A, Nisell R, Arborelius UP, Ekholm J. Varus and valgus loads on the knee joint during ergometer cycling. *Scand J Rehabil Med.* 1984;6:39-45.
26. Jorge M, Hull ML. Analysis of EMG measurements during bicycle pedaling. *J Biomech.* 1986;19:683-694.
27. Ericson MO, Bratt A, Nisell R, Arborelius UP, Ekholm J. Power output and work in different muscle groups during ergometer cycling. *Eur J Appl Physiol.* 1986;55:229-335.
28. Bosco C, Tarkka I, Komi PV. Effect of elastic energy and myoelectrical potentiation of triceps surae during stretch-shortening cycle exercise. *J Sports Med.* 1982;3:137-140.
29. Eisner WD, Bode SD, Nyland J, Caborn DNM. Electromyographic timing analysis of forward and backward cycling. *Med Sci Sports Exerc.* 1999;31:449-455.
30. Kautz SA, Hull ML. A theoretical basis for interpreting the force applied to the pedal in cycling. *J Biomech.* 1993;26:155-165.
31. Brown DA, Kautz SA, Dairaghi CA. Muscle activity patterns altered during pedaling at different body orientations. *J Biomech.* 1996;29:1349-1356.

SUGGESTED READINGS

Brand RA, Crowninshield RD, Johnston RC, Pedersen DR. Forces on the femoral head during activities of daily living. *Iowa Orthop J*. 1982;2:43-49.

Brown DA, Kautz SA. Increased workload enhances force output during pedaling exercise in person with poststroke hemiplegia. *Stroke*. 1998;29:598-606.

Brown DA, Kautz SA, Dairaghi CA. Muscle activity adapts to antigravity posture during pedaling in persons with poststroke hemiplegia. *Brain*. 1997;120:825-837.

Croft P, Cooper C, Wickham C, Coggon D. Osteoarthritis of the hip and occupational activity. *Scand J Work Environ Health*. 1992;18:59-63.

Holmes CJ, Pruitt AL, Whalen JJ. Iliotibial band syndrome in cyclists. *Am J Sports Med*. 1993;21:419-424.

Laubenthal KN, Smidt GL, Kettelkamp DB. A quantitative analysis of knee motion during activities of daily living. *Phys Ther*. 1972;52:34-42.

Lunnen YD, Yack J, LeVeau BF. Relationship between muscle length, muscle activity, and torque of the hamstring muscles. *Phys Ther*. 1981;61:190-195.

Marsch AP, Martin PE. The relationship between cadence and lower extremity EMG in cyclists and noncyclists. *Med Sci Sports Exerc*. 1995;27:217-225.

McLennan JG, McLennan JC. Cycling and the older athlete. *Sports Med in Older Athlete*. 1991;10:291-299.

Munnings F. Cyclist's palsy. *Phys & Sports Med*. 1991;19:113-119.

Nakayama DK, Gardner MJ, Rogers KD. Disability from bicycle related injuries in children. *J Trauma*. 1990;30:1390-1394.

Neptune RR, Kautz SA, Hull ML. The effect of pedaling rate on coordination in cycling. *J Biomech*. 1997;30:1051-1058.

Reilley DT, Martens M. Experimental analysis of the quadriceps muscle force and patellofemoral joint reaction force for various activities. *Acta Orthop Scand*. 1972;43:126-137.

Rosecrance JC, Giuliani CA. Kinematic analysis of lower limb movement during ergometer pedaling in hemiplegic and nonhemiplegic subjects. *Phys Ther*. 1991;71:334-343.

Suzuki S, Watanabe S, Homma S. EMG activity and kinematics of human cycling movements at different constant velocities. *Brain Res*. 1982;240:245-258.

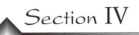

Section IV

Back Analyses

Donning a Shoe

INTRODUCTION AND SET-UP

People use various techniques to don and tie their shoes. Some individuals sit to don and tie their shoes; others sit to don and then stand to tie their shoes; while others stand to don and tie their shoes. This particular analysis focused on the activity of the back involved in putting on one's shoes.

Before proceeding with this analysis, a brief review of the anatomy of the spinal components is presented to enhance the reader's understanding of the muscular analysis. The joints involved in this analysis included the atlanto-occipital and atlantoaxial joints, the intervertebral joints, the facet joints of the spine, the sacroiliac joints, and the hip joints. In addition, the costovertebral and costotransverse joints were involved indirectly.

Spinal movement and stability is related to the characteristics of the vertebrae of each region of the spine (cervical versus thoracic versus lumbar).[1-4] The vertebral bodies are small in the cervical region, with uncinate processes posterolaterally that limit lateral motion. Relatively large vertebral discs and short, horizontally oriented spinous processes allow for great mobility of the intervertebral joints. Flexion of the upper segments consists of anterior tilting and posterior gliding, while extension of the lower segments consists of posterior tilting and anterior gliding. Lateral tilting and rotation are also possible. The superior and inferior facets glide and rotate. Their spatial orientations (superior facets face upward, backward, and medially; inferior facets face downward, forward, and laterally) permit flexion and extension while limiting rotation.[5-8]

Most of the flexion seen in the cervical region comes from the atlanto-occipital joint, where the skull articulates with C-1 (the atlas). Rotation comes from the atlantoaxial joint, where C-1 spins on the odontoid process of C-2 (the axis).[5-8]

In the thoracic region, the vertebral bodies are fairly uniform in shape, with demifacets for articulation with the ribs on the posterolateral aspects. The vertebral bodies and discs are larger than those seen in the cervical area. The intervertebral joints permit anterior tilting and posterior gliding during flexion, as well as lateral tilting and rotation. However, the oblique downward angle of the spinous processes makes flexion nearly impossible in the midthoracic area.[9]

Like the cervical facets, the thoracic facets glide and rotate. The superior facets face upward, backward, and laterally; the inferior facets face downward, forward, and medially. Flexion is limited by this arrangement. In addition, the costotransverse and costovertebral joints further restrict movement. These attachments help stabilize the spine while limiting movement.

The lumbar vertebrae are even larger than the thoracic vertebrae and somewhat block-shaped. The spinous processes are horizontally angled, which allows flexion to occur. The intervertebral joints permit anterior tilting and posterior gliding and make flexion, rotation, and lateral flexion possible. The superior facets face backward and medially, while the inferior facets face forward and laterally. The superior facets are concave, while the inferior facets are convex. This arrangement permits gliding and spinning to occur, which in turn accounts for the additional flexion mobility seen in the lumbar area.[10-13]

In addition to serving mobility, the vertebral discs serve as shock absorbers. With unsupported sitting, the load in the discs is increased to 40% compared to erect standing. When flexion and rotation are combined, the load is increased to 400%.[14-16]

The sacroiliac joints restrict movement and create stability in the sacral region.[17] The thoracolumbar fascia, which serves as muscular origin, acts as a support mechanism, or belt, as the muscle forces pull on the edges of the fascia.[18]

The anterior longitudinal ligament, running along the anterior aspect of the vertebral bodies, and the anterior atlantoaxial ligament limit extension as they become taut during this motion. The posterior longitudinal ligament, running along the posterior aspect of the vertebral bodies, and the tectorial membrane limit flexion as they become taut during flexion. The supraspinous ligament and the ligamentum nuchae traverse the tips of the spinous processes. The ligamentum flavum and the posterior atlantoaxial ligament run from lamina to lamina, and the interspinous ligament runs from one spinous process to another. These last five ligaments limit flexion as they become taut in flexion. Lateral flexion is limited by the contralateral intertransverse ligaments running from one transverse process to another.[2-3]

In addition, the lumbar spine is stabilized by the iliolumbar ligament, which runs from L-4 and L-5 to the anterior iliac crest. The sacrospinal and sacrotuberal ligaments help secure the pelvis and limit excessive anterior tilting as they traverse the posterior aspect of the pelvis. Finally, the sacroiliac joints are stabilized by the anterior and posterior sacroiliac ligaments.[2-3]

Although the composite motion of all vertebral segments provides a large range of motion, the hip joints contribute to the greater range of motion seen in the performance of ADL. This is due to the concept known as lumbopelvic rhythm. During the performance of ADLs, lumbopelvic rhythm permits the pelvis to tilt anteriorly, while the spine flexes forward, thereby increasing the range of motion seen.[19]

With this brief summary of factors that contribute to the mobility and stability of the spinal components completed, the muscular analysis can now proceed. The subject was seated in a chair with a seat height of 29 inches. The subject held the shoe in the contralateral hand. The subject was upright with the lower spine aligned in neutral and the head and neck flexed forward. The hip and knee joints were flexed 90 degrees, and the ankle joints were in neutral (Figure 12-1). In this activity, the thoracolumbar trunk flexed, and the neck extended in the lower segments while flexing in the upper segments. There was also lateral flexion and rotation present in all areas of the spine.

BRINGING THE TRUNK FORWARD

Starting in the upright sitting posture, the subject flexed the trunk forward to approximately 15 degrees (Figure 12-2). Concentric contraction of the rectus abdominis and internal abdominal obliques (both external and internal) caused this motion to occur. After the initial forward flexion, the trunk extensor muscles provided the primary force for completing the forward flexion. The eccentric contractions of the thoracic and lumbar erector spinae muscles primarily controlled the extent and rate of flexion as gravity pulled the trunk toward the floor. The semispinalis, multifidus, and rotatores muscles assisted the erector spinae muscles during this time.[20-26]

As the activity continued, the trunk continued flexing forward to approximately 70 degrees (Figure 12-3). The eccentric activity of the trunk extensors continued until approximately two-thirds of maximal flexion had been achieved. During this time, there was eccentric activity of the hip extensors (gluteus maximus and hamstring muscles), which helped to control the forward flexion of the trunk against gravity.[27]

Figure 12-1. Starting position: The subject was seated, holding the left shoe in the right hand. The key landmarks denoted by black dots are: A = acromion process (superior aspect); V = greater trochanter of femur; and W = spinous process of C-7.

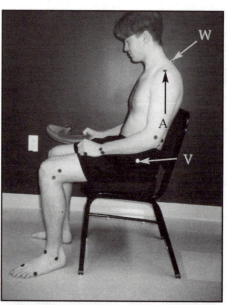

Figure 12-2. Bringing the trunk forward: The subject began to flex forward at the waist to bring the shoe toward the left foot. The key landmarks denoted by black dots are: A = acromion process (superior aspect); V = greater trochanter of femur; W = spinous process of C-7; X = spinous process of T-12; and Y = spinous process of L-5.

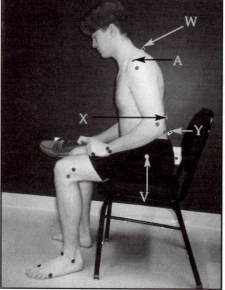

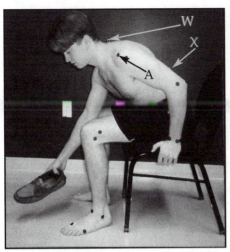

Figure 12-3. Bringing the trunk forward: The subject continued to flex forward to approximately 70 degrees. The lower cervical spine extended while the upper cervical spine flexed. The key landmarks denoted by black dots are: A = acromion process (superior aspect); W = spinous process of C-7; and X = spinous process of T-12.

While the subject flexed the trunk, there was need for a small degree of extension (26 degrees) of the lower cervical spine (C-3 through C-7) with a small amount of flexion (6 degrees) of the upper cervical spine (occiput through C-2), which enabled the subject to see the shoe. The extension component of the lower cervical spine was brought about by the concentric contractions of the trapezius, semispinalis capitis and cervicis, splenius capitis and cervicis, and the upper erector spinae muscles. The flexion component of the upper cervical spine was brought about by the concentric contractions of the sternocleidomastoid, rectus capitis lateralis, and rectus capitis anterior muscles.[27]

In addition, as the final degrees of trunk forward flexion were reached, there was a minimal amount of cervical rotation (8 degrees) needed to don the shoe, specifically enabling the subject to see the task being performed. In the cervical region, the rotation was accompanied by side flexion. This dual motion was due to the coronally oblique positions of the articular facet joints. In this particular activity, the rotation occurred primarily in the suboccipital region, and the lateral flexion was to the opposite side.[28]

The main muscle that produced this motion was the sternocleidomastoid muscle, contracting concentrically to produce a contralateral rotation of the cervical spine. Other muscles that assisted the sternocleidomastoid muscle were the multifidus, semispinalis capitis, rotatores and levatores muscles. All contracted concentrically to produce a contralateral rotation of the cervical spine.

In addition to the trunk forward flexion, 12 degrees of trunk rotation were needed to bring the contralateral arm toward the shoe (Figure 12-4).

Figure 12-4. Bringing the trunk forward: The subject rotated the trunk to the left to bring the contralateral arm toward the right shoe. The key landmarks denoted by black dots are: W = spinous process of C-7; X = spinous process of T-12; Y = spinous process of L-5; Z = rib angle; and AA = iliac crest (posterior aspect).

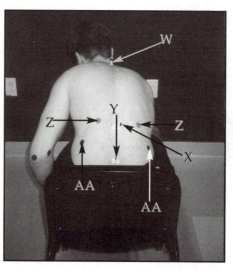

This rotation was brought about by the contralateral external and ipsilateral internal abdominal oblique muscles, contracting concentrically. The semispinalis, multifidus, rotatores, and latissimus dorsi muscles assisted with this trunk rotation. They worked concentrically to produce contralateral rotation of the trunk. In addition, these muscles helped to oppose the flexion effect of the abdominal muscles during spinal rotation.[29]

PLACING THE FOOT IN THE SHOE

In order to place the foot in the shoe, the subject had to elevate the pelvis and flex the hip joint approximately 5 degrees once the trunk was flexed forward enough (Figure 12-5). The quadratus lumborum and iliocostalis lumborum muscles concentrically contracted to elevate, or hike, the hip. To counterbalance the pull of these muscles, the external abdominal oblique, latissimus dorsi, and hip abductors muscles worked concentrically on the contralateral side. This countertorque prevented the subject from falling toward the unsupported side of the body. The hip flexed as a result of concentric activity of the iliopsoas muscle.[20, 22-24]

To complete donning the shoe, the subject simultaneously pushed down with the lower extremity while using the index finger to hold the back of the shoe in place, so the foot could be slid into the shoe (Figure 12-6). Isometric contractions of the abdominal muscles stabilized the ribs and pelvis, while the latissimus dorsi and gluteus maximus muscles

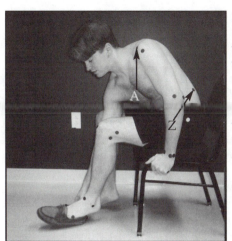

Figure 12-5. Placing the foot in the shoe: The subject flexed the left hip joint to place the foot in the shoe. The key landmarks denoted by black dots are: A = acromion process (superior aspect), V = greater trochanter of femur; and Z = rib angle.

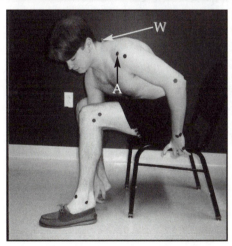

Figure 12-6. Placing the foot in the shoe: The subject held the back of the shoe steady while pushing the left lower extremity downward into the shoe. The key landmarks denoted by black dots are: A = acromion process (superior aspect) and W = spinous process of C-7.

helped to stabilize the vertebral column. The activity of these three muscles created an active tension in the thoracolumbar fascia, which assisted the erector spinae muscles in stabilization.[18]

SUMMARY

Key Landmarks for Shoe Analysis

Hip Complex: Greater trochanter of femur
                    Iliac crest (posterior aspect)

Spinal Complex: Spinous process of C-7
                    Spinous process of T-12
                    Spinous process of L-5
                    Rib angle

Shoulder Complex: Acromion process (superior aspect)

Major Phases for Shoe Analysis

Starting Position

• Position of subject

• Position of shoe

Bringing the Trunk Forward

Placing the Foot in the Shoe

Back Joint Motions and Muscular Activity: Donning a Shoe

Introduction and Set-Up

• Forward flexion of head and neck.

• Thoracolumbar spine in neutral.

Bringing the Trunk Forward

• Forward flexion and rotation to left of thoracolumbar spine.

• Extension of C-3 through C-7 spine.

• Flexion of occiput through C-2.

• Rotation to left with lateral flexion to right of suboccipital region.

• Primarily concentric muscular contractions of all muscles except eccentric muscular activity for muscles involved with forward flexion of thoracolumbar spine.

Placing the Foot in the Shoe

• Elevation of right pelvis and flexion of right hip joint via concentric muscular contractions.

• Thoracolumbar spine and suboccipital region maintain their positions via isometric muscular contractions.

CLINICAL APPLICATION AND DISCUSSION QUESTIONS

This particular analysis focused on the activity of the spinal components. Discuss the activity of the upper and lower extremities in completing this activity. Compare this analysis to one in which the subject stands to don the shoes. What differences would be seen in the upper extremity motions if a tie shoe was used?

Compare the motions of this activity to that of donning a pair of pants or tying shoelaces. How are the motions similar? How are they different?

What other activities are similar to the one presented in this analysis?

What types of assistive devices would be of value in an activity such as this? Why?

Finally, make a list of muscle substitutions for the prime movers of this analysis. Compare your list to Chart 3 in Appendix A.

REFERENCES

1. Gracovetsky S, Farfan H. The optimum spine. *Spine.* 1986;11:543-573.

2. Panjabi M, Abumi K, Duranceau J, Oxland T. Spinal stability and intersegmental muscle forces: a biomechanical model. *Spine.* 1989;14:194-200.

3. White AA, Panjabi MM. The basic kinematics of the human spine: a review of past and current knowledge. *Spine.* 1978;3:12-20.

4. White AA, Johnson RM, Panjabi MM, Southwick WO. Biomechanical analysis of clinical stability in the cervical spine. *Clin Orthop.* 1975;109:85-96.

5. Panjabi M, Dvorak J, Duranceau J, et al. Three-dimensional movements of the upper cervical spine. *Spine*. 1988;13:726-730.

6. Ålund M, Larsson SE. Three-dimensional analysis of neck motion: a clinical method. *Spine*. 1990;15:87-91.

7. Dimnet J, Pasquet A, Krag MH, Panjabi MM. Cervical spine motion in sagittal plane: kinematic and geometric parameters. *J Biomech*. 1982;12:959-969.

8. Penning L. Normal movements of the cervical spine. *American Journal of Roentgenology*. 1978;130:317-326.

9. Twomey LT, Taylor JR. Sagittal movements of the human vertebral column: a qualitative study of the role of the posterior vertebral elements. *Arch Phys Med Rehabil*. 1983;64:322-324.

10. Adams MA, Dolan P. Recent advances in lumbar spine mechanics and their clinical significance. *Clin Biomech*. 1995;10:3-19.

11. Battie MC, Bigos SJ, Sheehy A, Wortley MD. Spinal flexibility and individual factors that influence it. *Phys Ther*. 1987;67:653-657.

12. Koreska J, Robertston D, Milss RH, Gibson DA, Albisser AM. Biomechanics of the lumbar spine and its clinical significance. *Orthop Clin North Am*. 1977;8:121-133.

13. Thurston AJ, Harris JD. Normal kinematics of the lumbar spine and pelvis. *Spine*. 1983;8:199-205.

14. Jensen GM. Biomechanics of the lumbar intervertebral disk: a review. *Phys Ther*. 1980;60:4.

15. Nachemson AL. Disc pressure measurements. *Spine*. 1981;6:93-95.

16. Weihoffer SL, Guyer R, Herbert M, Griffith SL. Intradiscal pressure measurements above an instrumented fusion. *Spine*. 1995;20:516-530.

17. DonTigny RL. Function and pathomechanics of the sacroiliac joint: a review. *Phys Ther*. 1985;65:35-44.

18. Bogduk N, MacIntosh JE. The applied anatomy of the thoracolumbar fascia. *Spine*. 1984;9:164-170.

19. Cailliet R. *Soft Tissue Pain and Disability*. 2nd ed. Philadelphia, Pa: FA Davis Co; 1988.

20. Ladin Z, Murthy KK, DeLuca CJ. Mechanical recruitment of low-back muscles. *Spine*. 1989;14:927-938.

21. Bartelink DL. The role of abdominal pressure in relieving the pressure on the lumbar intervertebral disc. *J Bone Joint Surg Br*. 1957;39:718-725.

22. Carmon DJ, Blanton PL, Biggs NL. Electromyographic study of the anterolateral musculature utilizing indwelling electrodes. *Am J Phys Med*. 1972;51:113-129.

23. Floyd WF, Silver PHS. Function of the erectores spinae in flexion of the trunk. *Lancet*. 1951;260:133-134.

24. Floyd WF, Silver PHS. The function of the erectores spinae muscle in certain movements and postures in man. *J Physiol (Lond)*. 1955;129:184-203.

25. Strohl KP, Mead J, Banzett RB, Loring SH, Kosch PC. Regional differences in abdominal muscle activity during various maneuvers in humans. *J Appl Physiol*. 1981;51:1471-1476.

26. Walker ML, Rothstein JM, Finucane SD, Lamb RL. Relationships between lumbar lordosis, pelvic tilt, and abdominal muscle performance. *Phys Ther*. 1987;67:512-516.

27. Furlani J, Berzin F, Vitti M. Electromyographic study of the gluteus maximus muscle. *Electromyogr Clin Neurophysiol*. 1974;14:377-388.

28. Goel VK, Clark CR, Gallaes K, Liu YK. Moment-rotation relationships of the ligamentous occipito-atlantoaxial complex. *J Biomech*. 1988;8:673-680.

29. Kumar S, Narayan Y, Zedka M. An electromyographic study of unresisted trunk rotation with normal velocity among healthy subjects. *Spine*. 1996;21:1500-1512.

SUGGESTED READINGS

Adams MA, Hutton WC. Has the lumbar spine a margin of safety in forward bending? *Clin Biomech*. 1986;1:3-6.

Adams MAP, Dolan CM, Hutton WC. An electronic inclinometer technique for measuring lumbar curvature. *Clin Biomech*. 1986;1:130-134.

Baolgun JA, Abereoje OK, Olaogun MO, Obajuluwa VA. Inter- and intratester reliability of measuring neck motions with tape measure and Myrin gravity reference goniometer. *J Orthop Sports Phys Ther*. 1989;10:248-253.

Bogduk N. A reappraisal of the anatomy of the human lumbar erector spinae. *J Anat*. 1980;131:525-540.

Burton AK. Regional lumbar sagittal mobility: measurement by flexicurves. *Clin Biomed*. 1986;1:20-26.

Bustami FM. A new description of the lumbar erector spinae muscle in man. *J Anat*. 1986;144:81-91.

Chari VR, Kirby RL. Lower-limb influence on sitting balance while reaching forward. *Arch Phys Med Rehabil*. 1986;67:730-733.

Fielding JW. Cineroentgenography of the normal cervical spine. *J Bone Joint Surg Am*. 1957;39:1280-1288.

Fraser EJ. Extensor muscle of the low back: an electromyographic study. *Phys Ther*. 1967;47:200-207.

Madson TJ, Youdas JW, Suman VJ. Reproducibility of lumbar spine range of motion measurements using the back range of motion device. *J Orthop Sports Phys Ther*. 1999;29:470-477.

Mayer TG, Kondraske G, Beals SB, Gatchel RJ. Spinal range of motion: accuracy and sources of error with inclinometric measurement. *Spine*. 1997;22:1976-1984.

Merritt JL, McLean TJ, Erichson RP, Offord KP. Measurement of trunk flexibility in normal subjects: reproducibility of three clinical methods. *Mayo Clin Proc.* 1986;61:192-197.

Moroney SP, Schultz AB, Miller JA. Analysis and measurement of loads on the neck. *J Orthop Res.* 1988;6:713-720.

Nolan JP, Sherk HH. Biomechanical evaluation of the extensor musculature of the cervical spine. *Spine.* 1988;13:9-11.

Panjabi M. Symposium on the lumbar spine. *Orthop Clin North Am.* 1977;8:169-179.

Panjabi MM, Krag MH, Goel VK. A technique for measurement and description of three-dimensional six-degree-of-freedom motion of a body joint with an application to the human spine. *J Biomech.* 1981;14:447-460.

Panjabi MM, Oxland TR, Yamamoto I, Crisco JJ. Mechanical behavior of the human lumbar and lumbosacral spine as shown by three-dimensional load-displacement curves. *J Bone Joint Surg Am.* 1994;76:413-424.

Pearcy MJ, Gill JM, Whittle MW, Johnson GR. Dynamic back movement measured using a three-dimensional television system. *J Biomech.* 1987;20:943-949.

Pearcy MJ, Hindle RJ. New method for the non-invasive three-dimensional measurement of human back movement. *Clin Biomech.* 1989;4:73-79.

Rheault W, Ferris S, Foley JA, Schaffhauser D, Smith R. Intertester reliability of the flexible ruler for the cervical spine. *J Orthop Sports Phys Ther.* 1989;10:254-256.

VanKuyk-Minis MAH. Assistive devices: integral to the daily lives of human beings. *Clin Rheumatol.* 1998;17:3-5.

Youdas JW, Carey JR, Garrett TR. Reliability of measurements of cervical spine range of motion—comparison of three methods. *Phys Ther.* 1991;71:98-104.

Youdas JW, Suman VJ, Garrett TR. Reliability of measurements of lumbar spine sagittal mobility obtained with the flexible curve. *J Orthop Sports Phys Ther.* 1995;21:13-20.

Chapter 13

Lifting a Package From the Trunk of a Car

INTRODUCTION AND SET-UP

Loads ranging from a few pounds to 50+ pounds are lifted on a daily basis: parents lift babies in and out of cribs; individuals lift and lower objects to kitchen countertops and in and out of refrigerators; others move packages in and out of car trunks. The back complex plays an important role in activities such as these. The vertebral column is stabilized by the joint structure itself, as well as by muscles and ligaments. Although the ligaments help support and stabilize the vertebral column, the muscles provide the greater support and stabilization.[1-8] Improper body mechanics can cause injury to the lower back during an activity such as lifting.

This analysis focused on lifting a 50-pound bag of fertilizer from the trunk of a car and carrying the bag to and placing it down on a shelf. The shelf was 24 inches off the ground. Proper body mechanics were maintained. This included lifting in a symmetrical pattern in a sagittal plane, keeping the center of the object as close to the body as possible, bending the knees to decrease the stress of the line of gravity, lifting slowly, not twisting the trunk, and maintaining a lumbar lordosis.[9-16]

MOVING THE BODY TOWARD THE PACKAGE

The analysis started with the subject standing in back of the car and facing the trunk, which was already opened. The opening of the trunk was an ergonomic design, which meant that the center portion was cut out for greater ease in moving objects in and out of the trunk. The bag to be lifted was 18 inches from the subject and 15 inches from the ground (Figure 13-1). From this position, the subject moved the right lower extremity forward and flexed forward at the hip joints, while flexing the knee joints.

Figure 13-1. Starting position: The subject is standing in front of the open trunk of the car. The trunk has an ergonomic opening. The key landmarks denoted by black dots are: W = spinous process of C-7; X = spinous process of T-12; and Z = rib angle.

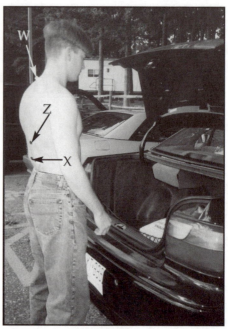

The hips were flexed 40 degrees and the knees, 35 degrees. The back was maintained in its normal lordotic position[17] (Figure 13-2).

The iliopsoas muscles worked concentrically to initiate hip flexion, while the quadriceps femoris muscles worked eccentrically to control knee flexion. The abdominal muscles, in tandem with the iliopsoas muscles, worked concentrically, which created the initial forward motion of the trunk. However, the erector spinae, gluteus maximus, and quadratus lumborum muscles worked eccentrically to control the forward flexion of the hip joints once the trunk passed anterior to the lower extremities.[18-24]

Once the subject grasped the package, it was slid toward the subject (Figure 13-3) in order to enable him to get a better grip on the package prior to lifting. The trunk and lower extremities maintained their previous positions through isometric contractions of the muscles cited above.

LIFTING THE PACKAGE

Once in position, the subject lifted the load (Figure 13-4) and returned to the starting position. The motions were the exact opposite of the forward bending. The quadriceps femoris and gluteus maximus muscles worked concentrically to bring the body to an upright position.

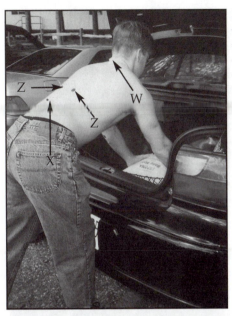

Figure 13-2. Moving the body toward the package: The subject flexed the hip and knee joints as the trunk and upper extremities were moved toward the package. The key landmarks denoted by black dots are: W = spinous process of C-7; X = spinous process of T-12; and Z = rib angle.

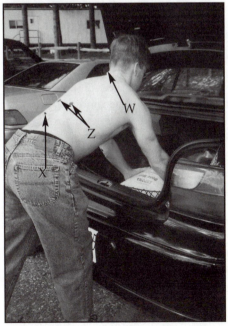

Figure 13-3. Moving the package closer to the subject: The subject slid the package closer to himself while maintaining his trunk and lower extremity positions. The key landmarks denoted by black dots are: W = spinous process of C-7; X = spinous process of T-12; and Z = rib angle.

Figure 13-4. Lifting the package: The subject used the lower extremities to push the superimposed body weight upward. The back was maintained in an erect posture. The key landmarks denoted by black dots are: W = spinous process of C-7; X = spinous process of T-12; and Z = rib angle.

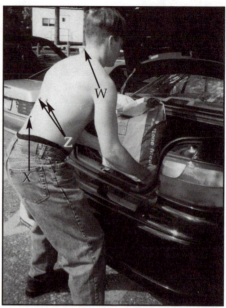

The abdominal muscles worked isometrically, while the erector spinae muscles worked concentrically to keep the vertebral column properly positioned during the lift.[7] The quadratus lumborum muscles worked isometrically to provide stabilization. Once upright (Figure 13-5), the muscles of the back worked isometrically to control posture as the muscular activity of the lower extremities produced the gait motions, and the muscular activity of the upper extremities supported the load being carried.[24-37]

PLACING THE PACKAGE ON A SHELF

As the subject began to place the load on the shelf (Figure 13-6), the hip and knee joints were flexed to lower the body to the correct height. The hips flexed 55 degrees and the knees, 30 degrees. Once again, the back was maintained in a normal lordotic curve. The muscular activity was the same as described for the activity needed to position the subject in order to be able to lift the load. However, there was increased muscular activity due to the superimposed weight of the package.[18-24]

When standing upright, the forces acting on the vertebral column were in a vertical direction. As the subject flexed forward, the weight of the upper body came to lie parallel to the disc-body junction of the vertebral column, creating a shearing force on the disc-body junction.

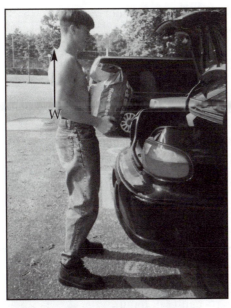

Figure 13-5. Upright posture to carry the package to the shelf: The subject maintained an erect trunk, bringing the package close to the body for carrying. The key landmark denoted by the black dot is W = spinous process of C-7.

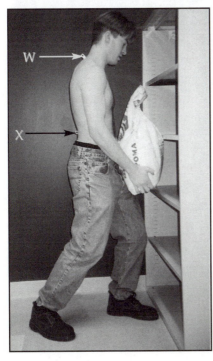

Figure 13-6. Placing the package on the shelf: The subject flexed the hip and knee joints to lower the upper body and the package to the shelf prior to placing it on the shelf. The key landmarks denoted by black dots are: W = spinous process of C-7 and X = spinous process of T-12.

This caused the two sides of the posterior facet joints to compress each other and prevent significant shearing forces from developing on the disc itself. During forward flexion, the ligamentous system of the vertebral column was acted upon by muscular contractions of the abdominal, such as the transverse abdominals tensing the thoracolumbar fascia, which, in turn, pulled on the spinous processes. These indirect controls provided stabilization of the vertebral column and protected the disc from injury.[36-43]

In addition, the abdominal and thoracic cavities, being acted upon by muscular contractions, helped to transmit forces imposed on the spine, further taking pressure off the spine and helping to stabilize the spine.[24-27,41,43-44]

SUMMARY

Key Anatomical Landmarks for Lifting Analysis

Hip Complex: Greater trochanter of femur
                      Iliac crest

Spinal Complex: Spinous process of C-7
                      Spinous process of T-12
                      Spinous process of L-5
                      Rib angle

Major Phases for Lifting Analysis

Starting Position

• Position of subject

• Position of object to be lifted

Moving the Body Toward the Package

Lifting the Package

Placing the Package on the Shelf

Back Joint Motions and Muscular Activity: Lifting a Package From the Trunk of a Car

Introduction and Set-Up
- Forward flexion of head and neck.

- Thoracolumbar spine in neutral.

Moving the Body Toward the Package
- Primarily flexion of hip joints via concentric muscular activity.

- Eccentric activity of trunk muscles to control forward movement of trunk.

Lifting the Package
- Primarily extension of hip joints via concentric muscular activity.

- Thoracolumbar spine is maintaining position.

Placing the Package on a Shelf
- Primarily flexion of hip joints via concentric muscular contraction.

- Thoracolumbar spine is maintaining position.

CLINICAL APPLICATION AND DISCUSSION QUESTIONS

Proper body mechanics are a key factor in injury-free lifting. What are the key factors in proper body mechanics when lifting?

Ergonomically designed trunks on cars also assist individuals in lifting items from their cars. The newer ergonomic trunk designs allow the load to be slid closer to the individual prior to lifting, thus reducing the strain on the individual.

Think about the size of a package being moved, as well as the weight of the package. How will these two factors affect motion and muscular activity during lifting? What effect will sharing the load with another individual have on the muscular activity?

Think about the motions and the muscular activity of the cervical region of the spine in an activity such as this. How does it compare to the cervical analysis presented in the last chapter?

What motions and muscle activity would be seen in the upper extremities during this activity?

How will the size and weight of the package being lifted affect the upper extremity analysis? How would this analysis change if an older type trunk opening were used?

What other means could be used to lift a heavy package from a car trunk or from a shelf? (Hint: Think about the cranes used in industry.) What else could be done if these means were unavailable?

What roles do support belts play in lifting?

Lastly, what muscles could be substituted for the muscles cited in this analysis? Compare your muscle substitutions to those listed in Chart 3 in Appendix A.

REFERENCES

1. Gracovetsky S, Farfan H. The optimum spine. *Spine*. 1986;11:53-57.

2. Panjabi M, Abumi K, Duranceau J, Oxland T. Spinal stability and interseg-mental muscle forces: a biomechanical model. *Spine*. 1989;14:194-200.

3. White AA, Panjabi MM. The basic kinematics of the human spine: a review of past and current knowledge. *Spine*. 1978;3:12-20.

4. Buseck M, Schipplein OD, Andersson GB, Andriacchi TP. Influence of dynamic factors and external loads on the moment at the lumbar spine in lifting. *Spine*. 1988;13:918-921.

5. Sullivan MS. Back support mechanisms during manual lifting. *Phys Ther*. 1989;69:52-59.

6. Klausen K. The form and function of the loaded human spine. *Acta Physiol Scand*. 1965;65:176-190.

7. Morris JM, Lucas DB, Bresler B. Role of trunk in stability of the spine. *J Bone Joint Surg Am*. 1961;42:327-351.

8. Morris JM. Biomechanics of the spine. *Arch Surg*. 1973;107:418-423.

9. Chaffin DB, Baker W. A biomechanical model for analysis of symmetric sagittal plane lifting. *Trans Am Inst Indust Eng*. 1970;2:16-27.

10. Davies BT. Training in manual handling and lifting. In: Drury CG, ed. *Safety in Manual Materials Handling*. Cincinnati, Ohio: NIOSH;1978:175-178.

11. El-Bassoussi MM. *A dynamic biomechanical model for lifting in the sagittal plane*. Lubbock, Tex: Texas Tech University; 1974. Dissertation.

12. Freivalds A, Chaffin DB, Garg A, Lee KS. A dynamic biomechanical evalu-ation of lifting maximum acceptable loads. *J Biomech*. 1984;17:251-262.

13. Garg A. Evaluation of the NIOSH guidelines for manual lifting with special reference to horizontal distance. *Am Ind Hyg Assoc J.* 1989;50:157-164.

14. NIOSH. *A Work Practices Guide for Manual Lifting.* Cincinnati, Ohio: National Institute for Occupational Safety and Health; 1981. U.S. Dept. of Health and Human Services (NIOSH) technical report 81-122.

15. Snook SH. The design of manual handling tasks. *Ergonomics.* 1978;21:963-985.

16. Nordin M, Ortengren R, Andersson GBJ. Measurements of trunk movements during work. *Spine.* 1984;9:465-469.

17. Anderson CK, Chaffin DB, Herrin GD, Matthews LS. A biomechanical model of the lumbosacral joint during lifting activities. *J Biomech.* 1985;18:571-584.

18. Carlsöö S. The static muscle load in different work positions: an electromyographic study. *Ergonomics.* 1961;4:193-211.

19. Dolan P, Adams MA. The relationship between EMG activity and extensor moment generation in the erector spinae muscles during bending and lifting activities. *J Biomech.* 1993;26:513-522.

20. Floyd WF, Silver PHS. The function of the erectores spinae muscles in certain movements and postures in man. *J Physiol.* 1955;129:184-203.

21. Gracovetsky S, Kary M, Levy S, et al. Analysis of spinal and muscular activity during flexion/extension and free lifts. *Spine.* 90;15:1333-1339.

22. Tanii K, Masuda T. A kinesiological study of erectores spinae activity during trunk flexion and extension. *Ergonomics.* 1985;28:883-893.

23. Furlani J, Berzin F, Vitti M. Electromyographic study of the gluteus maximus muscle. *Electromyogr Clin Neurophysiol.* 1974;14:377-388.

24. Andersson GBJ, Ortengren R, Nachemson A. Intradiskal pressure, intraabdominal pressure, and myoelectric back muscle activity related to posture and loading. *Clin Orthop.* 1977;129:156-164.

25. Bartelink DL. The role of abdominal pressure in relieving the pressure on the lumbar intervertebral discs. *J Bone Joint Surg Br.* 1957;39:718-725.

26. Bearn JG. The significance of the activity of the abdominal muscles in weight lifting. *Acta Anat (BASEL).* 1961;45:83-89.

27. Floyd WF, Silver PHS. Electromyographic study of patterns of activity of the anterior abdominal wall muscles in man. *J Anat.* 1950;84:132-145.

28. Garg A. A comparison of isometric strength and dynamic lifting capability. *Ergonomics.* 1980;23:13-27.

29. Marras WS. Trunk motion during lifting: temporal relations among loading factors. *International Journal of Industrial Ergonomics.* 1987;1:159-167.

30. Svensson OK, Nemeth G, Ekholm H. Relative mechanical load on back and hip muscles during standing manual materials handling. *Scand J Rehabil Med.* 1987;19:179-186.

31. Zetterberg C, Andersson GBJ, Schultz AB. The activity of individual trunk muscles during heavy physical loading. *Spine.* 1987;12:1035-1040.

32. Joseph J, McColl I. Electromyography of muscles of posture: posterior vertebral muscles in males. *J Physiol (London)*. 1961;157:33-37.

33. Walker ML, Rothstein JM, Finucane SD, Lamb RL. Relationships between lumbar lordosis, pelvic tilt, and abdominal muscle performance. *Phys Ther*. 1987;67:512-516.

34. Nisell R. Mechanics of the knee: a study of joint and muscle load with clinical applications. *Acta Orthop Scand*. 1985;56:1-41.

35. Granta KP, Marras WS. The influence of trunk muscle coactivity on dynamic spinal loads. *Spine*. 1995;20:913-919.

36. Adams MA, Hutton WC. The effect of posture on the role of the apophyseal joints in resisting intervertebral compressive forces. *J Bone Joint Surg Br*. 1980;62:358-362.

37. Bogduk B, MacIntosh JE. The applied anatomy of thoracolumbar fascia. *Spine*. 1984;9:164-170.

38. Ekholm J, Arborelius UP, Nemeth G. The load on the lumbosacral joint and trunk muscle activity during lifting. *Ergonomics*. 1982;25:145-161.

39. Leskinen TPJ, Stalhammar HR, Kourinka JAA. A dynamic analysis of spinal compression with different lifting techniques. *Ergonomics*. 1983;26:595-604.

40. Shirazi-Adl A, Dronin G. Load-sharing function of lumbar intervertebral disc and facet joints in compression, extension, and flexion. *Advances in Bioengineering*. 1986;2:18-19.

41. Eie N, Wehn P. Measurement of the intra-abdominal pressure in relation to weight bearing of the lumbosacral spine. *Journal of the Oslo City Hospitals*. 1962;12:205-217.

42. Nachemson A. The load on lumbar discs in different positions of the body. *Clin Orthop*. 1966;45:107-122.

43. Strohl KP, Mead J, Banzett RB, Loring SH, Kosch PC. Regional differences in abdominal muscle activity during various maneuvers in humans. *J Appl Physiol*. 1981;51:1471-1476.

44. Nachemson AL. Disc pressure measurements. *Spine*. 1981;6:93-95.

SUGGESTED READINGS

Andersson GBJ, Ortengren R, Herberts P. Quantitative electromyographic studies of back muscle activity related to posture and loading. *Orthop Clin North Am*. 1977;8:85-96.

Andersson GBJ, Ortengren R, Schultz AB. Analysis and measurement of the loads on the lumbar spine during work at a table. *J Biomech*. 1980;13:513-520.

Bearn JG. An electromyographic study of the trapezius, deltoid, pectoralis major, biceps, and triceps muscles during static loading of the upper limb. *Anatomical Record*. 1961;140:103-108.

Bendix T, Eid SE. The distance between the load and the body with three bimanual lifting techniques. *Appl Ergonomics*. 1983;14:185-192.

Brown JR. Factors contributing to the development of low back pain in industrial workers. *Am Ind Hyg Assoc J*. 1975;36:26-31.

Bustami FM. A new description of the lumbar erector spinae muscle in man. *J Anat*. 1986;144:81-91.

Carlsöö S. A back and lift test. *Appl Ergonomics*. 1980;11:66-72.

Carlsöö S. Influence of frontal and dorsal loads on muscle activity and on the weight distribution in the feet. *Acta Orthop Scand*. 1964;34:299-309.

Carlsöö S. The static muscle load in different work positions: an electromyographic study. *Ergonomics*. 1961;4:193-211.

Chaffin DB, Park KS. A longitudinal study of low back pain as associated with occupational weight lifting factors. *Am Ind Hyg Assoc J*. 1973;34:513-525.

Davis PR, Stubbs DA. Safe levels of manual forces for young males (1). *Appl Ergonomics*. 1977;8:141-150.

Davis PR, Stubbs DA. Safe levels of manual forces for young males (2). *Appl Ergonomics*. 1977;8:219-228.

Davis PR, Stubbs DA. Safe levels of manual forces for young males (3). *Appl Ergonomics*. 1978;9:33-37.

Davis PR, Troup JDG, Burnard JH. Movements of the thoracic and lumbar spine when lifting: a chronocyclophotographic study. *J Anat (London)*. 1965;99:13-26.

Deusinger RH, Rose SJ. Analysis of external oblique EMG activity during back extension. *Phys Ther*. 1985;65:673-674.

Drury CG, Begbie K, Ulate C, Deeb JM. Experiments on wrist deviation in manual materials handling. *Ergonomics*. 1985;28:577-589.

Eie N. Load capacity of the low back. *Journal of the Oslo City Hospitals*. 1966;16:73-98.

Farfan HF. Muscular mechanisms of the lumbar spine and the position of power and efficiency. *Orthop Clin North Am*. 1975;6:135-144.

Gallagher S, Marras WS, Bobick TG. Lifting in stooped and kneeling postures: effects on lifting capacity, metabolic costs, and electromyography of eight trunk muscles. *International Journal of Industrial Ergonomics*. 1988;3:65-76.

Garg A, Ayoub MM. What criteria exist for determining how much load can be lifted? *Hum Factors*. 1980;22:475-486.

Garg A, Owen B. Reducing back stress to nursing personnel. *Ergonomics*. 1992;35:1353-1375.

Grieve DW. The dynamics of lifting. *Exerc Sport Sci Rev*. 1977;5:157-179.

Guthrie DI. A new approach to handling in industry. *S Afr Med J*. 1963;37:651-655.

Jorgensen K. Back muscle strength and body weight as limiting factors for work in standing slightly-stooped position. *Scand J Rehabil Med*. 1970;2:149-153.

Kippers V, Parker AW. Hand positions at possible critical points in the stoop-lift movement. *Ergonomics*. 1983;26:895-903.

Kumar S. Physiological responses to weight lifting in different planes. *Ergonomics*. 1980;23:987-993.

Kumar S, Davis PR. Interrelationship of physiological and biomechanical parameters during stoop lifting. *The International Congress of Physical Activity Sciences (Quebec)*. 1976;222.

Kumar S, Scaife WGS. A precision task, posture, and strain. *Journal of Safety Rescue*. 1979;11:28-36.

Legg SJ. The effect of abdominal muscle fatigue and training on the intra-abdominal pressure developed during lifting. *Ergonomics*. 1981;24:191-195.

Moroney SP, Schultz AB, Miller JA. Analysis and measurement of loads on the neck. *J Orthop Res*. 1988;6:713-720.

Panjabi M, Yamamoto I, Oxland T, Crisco J. How does posture affect coupling in the lumbar spine? *Spine*. 1989;14:1002-1011.

Panjabi MM, Oxland TR, Yamamoto I, Crisco JJ. Mechanical behavior of the human lumbar and lumbosacral spine as shown by three-dimensional load-displacement curves. *J Bone Joint Surg Am*. 1994;76:413-424.

Park KS, Chaffin DB. A biomechanical evaluation of two methods of manual load lifting. *Transactions of the American Institute of Industrial Engineers*. 1974;6:105-113.

Parnianpour M, Nordin M, Kahanovitz N, Frankel V. The triaxial coupling of torque generation of trunk muscles during isometric exertions and the effect of fatiguing isoinertial moments on the motor output and movement patterns. *Spine*. 1988;13:982-990.

Pearcy MJ. Twisting mobility of the human back in flexed postures. *Spine*. 1993;18:114-119.

Petersen CM, Amundsen LR, Schendel MJ. Comparison of the effectiveness of two pelvic stabilization systems on pelvic movement during maximal isometric trunk extension and flexion muscle contractions. *Phys Ther*. 1987;67:534-539.

Poulsen E. Back muscle strength and weight limits in lifting burdens. *Spine*. 1981;6:73-75.

Poulsen E, Jorgensen K. Back muscle strength, lifting, and stooped working postures. *Appl Ergonomics*. 1971;2:133-137.

Schultz AB, Andersson GBJ, Haderspeck K, Ortengren R, Nordin M, Bjork R. Analysis and measurement of lumbar trunk loads in tasks involving bends and twists. *J Biomech*. 1982;15:669-675.

Snijders CJ, Hoek van Dijke GA, Roosch ER. A biomechanical model for the analysis of the cervical spine in static postures. *J Biomech*. 1991;24:783-792.

Svensson OK, Arborelius UP, Ekholm J. Relative mechanical load on shoulder and elbow muscles in standing position when handling materials manually. *Scand J Rehabil Med*. 1987;19:169-178.

Troup JDG. Biomechanics of the vertebral column. Its application to prevention of back pain in the population and to assessment of working capacity in patients with lumbar spinal disability. *Physiother.* 1979;65:238-244.

Vulcan AP, King AI, Nakamura GS. Effects of bending on the vertebral column during +Gz acceleration. *Aerospace Medicine.* 1970;41:294-300.

Whitney RJ. The stability provided by the feet during maneuvers whilst standing. *J Anat.* 1962;96.103-111.

Yates JW, Kamon E, Rodgers SH, Champney PC. Static lifting strength and maximal isometric voluntary contractions of back, arm, and shoulder muscles. *Ergonomics.* 1980;23:37-47.

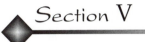

Upper and Lower Extremity Analysis

Chapter 14

Driving a Car

INTRODUCTION AND SET-UP

The act of driving a car is influenced by seat height, seat angle, seat distance from the pedals, type of car driven, type of transmission (manual versus automatic), and how an individual uses their feet to work the pedals of the car (toes versus entire foot; heel on floor versus heel off floor).[1-14]

This particular analysis covered the activities of both the upper and lower extremities. The focus was on the use of an automatic transmission and covered the biomechanics involved from a starting position in which both feet were resting on the floor, the left upper extremity was resting on the steering wheel at approximately the 10 o'clock position (using the face of a clock as the subject faced the wheel), and the right upper extremity was on the key, which was already in the ignition (Figure 14-1).

For purposes of this analysis, a training car at a rehabilitation facility was used. Therefore, the car was not actually driven on city streets in order to ensure safety when taking measurements. However, a simulation of the subject starting the car, driving for two city blocks, and then coming to a stop was performed. The simulated speed driven was 25 miles per hour, which is allowed in most residential neighborhoods.[15] The seat height was 17.5 inches with an angle of 103 degrees. The distance from the seat to the gas pedal was 132 inches, and the distance from the seat to the brake pedal, 119 inches. The ignition slot was located on the side of the drive shaft, 1 inch below the bottom of the gearshift. The gearshift was 2.75 inches anterior to the steering wheel.

The first part of this analysis focused on the activities of the upper extremities and was divided into several phases for ease of understanding: phase 1 covered the starting position for starting the engine; phase 2 covered moving from park to drive; phase 3 covered steering the car; phase 4 covered slowing down the car; and phase 5 covered applying the brake.

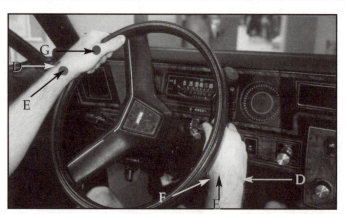

Figure 14-1. Starting positions of the upper extremities: The left hand was on the steering wheel at the 10 o'clock position. The right hand was on the key in the ignition. The key landmarks denoted by black dots are: D = ulnar head (dorsal aspect); E = radial styloid process (dorsal aspect); F = radial styloid process (radial aspect); and G = first MCP joint line.

The second part of this analysis focused on the activities of the lower extremities and was divided into similar phases: phase 1 covered starting the engine; phase 2, accelerating the car; phase 3, increasing the speed; phase 4, slowing down the car; and phase 5, applying the brake.

The third part of this analysis compared driving an automatic transmission to driving a manual transmission.

PART 1: UPPER EXTREMITY ANALYSIS WITH AUTOMATIC TRANSMISSION

Starting the Engine

Beginning in the position outlined in the introduction, the right upper extremity was in 45 degrees of shoulder forward flexion and 10 degrees of abduction. The elbow joint was flexed 45 degrees, and the forearm was pronated 70 degrees. The wrist joint was radially deviated 15 degrees. The hand was using a lateral prehension-type grip to grasp the key[16] (see Figure 14-1). The CMC joint of the thumb was flexed 8 degrees; the MCP joint, 34 degrees; and the IP joint was in neutral. The MCP joints of digits two through five were flexed 45, 40, 90, and 95 degrees, respectively.

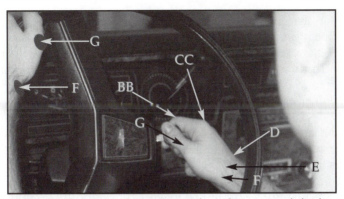

Figure 14-2. Starting the ignition: The subject turned the key half way, maintaining the lateral prehension grip on the key. The key landmarks denoted by black dots are: D = ulnar head (dorsal aspect); E = radial styloid process (dorsal aspect); F = radial styloid process (radial aspect); G = first MCP joint line; BB = PIP joint line; and CC = MCP joint line.

The PIP joints were flexed 60, 90, 95, and 105 degrees, respectively. The DIP joints of digits two through five were flexed 5, 35, 35, and 40 degrees, respectively.

As the key was turned halfway anteriorly (Figure 14-2), the shoulder joint maintained its original position. The elbow joint flexed an additional 5 degrees, and the forearm was supinated 30 degrees, bringing the forearm to 40 degrees of pronation. The wrist joint was flexed 5 degrees. The wrist joint was also ulnarly deviated 35 degrees, bringing it to 20 degrees of ulnar deviation. The positions of the digits remained the same.

From a muscular perspective, there was an interplay between isometric activity and concentric activity to operate the car. In the initial key turning aspect, the right shoulder muscles (upper and lower trapezius, serratus anterior, levator scapulae, anterior deltoid, supraspinatus, and coracobrachialis) worked isometrically to maintain the shoulder position.[17-18] The biceps brachii, brachialis, and brachioradialis worked concentrically to control the elbow motion. The supinator and biceps brachii muscles worked concentrically to control the forearm position.[19-21] The flexors carpi ulnaris and radialis muscles worked concentrically at the wrist joint, with the flexor carpi ulnaris having the greater contribution due to the ulnar deviation needed at this time.[22] The muscles of the digits (flexors pollicis longus and brevis, flexors digitorum superficialis and profundus, flexor digiti minimi, lumbricals, and interossei) all worked isometrically to maintain the grasp on the key.[23-25]

To start the ignition, the key was turned completely anteriorly (Figure 14-3). Once again, the shoulder joint maintained its original position. The elbow joint extended 5 degrees, bringing the elbow joint to 45 degrees of flexion. The forearm was supinated an additional 5 degrees, bringing the forearm to 35 degrees of pronation. The wrist joint was flexed an additional 3 degrees, bringing it to 38 degrees of flexion. The wrist joint was ulnarly deviated an additional 5 degrees, bringing it to 25 degrees of ulnar deviation. The position of the digits had not changed.

To complete the turning of the key, the shoulder musculature continued its isometric work. The triceps brachii and anconeus muscles worked concentrically to extend the elbow.[26-27] The supinator and biceps brachii muscles continued to work concentrically to supinate the forearm. The wrist flexors also continued their concentric activity, with the flexor carpi ulnaris muscle contributing more to the activity due to the continuing ulnar deviation. The muscles of the digits continued isometrically to maintain the grasp on the key.

During this entire procedure, the left upper extremity remained in position on the steering wheel (see Figure 14-3). The shoulder joint was in 50 degrees of flexion and the elbow joint in 105 degrees of flexion. The forearm was in 45 degrees of pronation and the wrist joint in 25 degrees of ulnar deviation. The hand maintained a cylindrical grip on the wheel. All the joints of digits two through five were in varying degrees of flexion. The MCP joints, from two to five, were flexed 35, 50, 62, and 75 degrees, respectively. The PIP joints were flexed 60, 75, 75, and 55 degrees, respectively, and the DIP joints were flexed 35, 45, 30, and 17 degrees, respectively. The thumb was held in neutral, resting against the wheel.

During this entire time, the muscles of the left upper extremity worked isometrically to maintain the position of the left upper extremity on the wheel. The upper and lower trapezius, serratus anterior, latissimus dorsi, anterior deltoid, supraspinatus, and coracobrachialis muscles were active at the shoulder joint.[17-18] The biceps brachii and brachialis muscles were active at the elbow joint. The pronators teres and quadratus muscles controlled the forearm position.[19-21] The flexor carpi ulnaris and the extensor carpi ulnaris muscles controlled the wrist position.[22] The flexor digitorum profundus muscles maintained the position of the digits.[23-25]

Moving the Right Upper Extremity to the Gearshift

Once the ignition was started, the right upper extremity moved from the keys to the gearshift to engage it in the drive position (Figure 14-4).

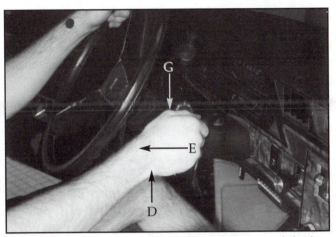

Figure 14-3. Starting the ignition: The subject turned the key completely forward, maintaining the grip on the key. The key landmarks denoted by black dots are: D = ulnar head (dorsal aspect); E = radial styloid process (dorsal aspect); and G = MCP joint line.

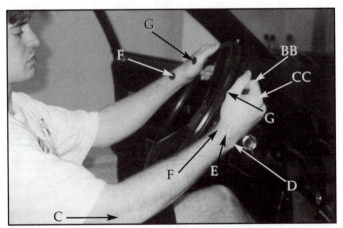

Figure 14-4. Moving the right upper extremity to the gear shift: The subject used a cylindrical grip to grasp the gear shift. The key landmarks denoted by black dots are: C = lateral epicondyle of humerus; D = ulnar head (dorsal aspect); E = radial styloid process (dorsal aspect); F = radial styloid process (radial aspect); G = first MCP joint line; BB = PIP joint line; and CC = MCP joint line.

The shoulder joint flexed an additional 5 degrees, bringing the shoulder joint to 50 degrees of flexion. The elbow joint flexed an additional 25 degrees, bringing the elbow joint to 70 degrees of flexion. The forearm supinated 45 degrees, bringing the forearm to 5 degrees of supination. The wrist joint flexed an additional 7 degrees and radially deviated 35 degrees. This brought the wrist joint to 45 degrees of flexion and 10 degrees of radial deviation. The joints of all the digits extended 25 degrees to release the grip on the key and then flexed to grasp the gearshift. However, the thumb remained in the extended position as it was brought into opposition with the index finger as the hand formed a cylindrical grip around the gearshift. The MCP joints of digits two to five flexed 50, 90, 95, and 105 degrees, respectively. The PIP joints of these digits flexed 45, 90, 95, and 100 degrees, respectively. The DIP joints flexed 10, 45, 45, and 45 degrees, respectively. As the shoulder and elbow joints extended an additional 5 degrees each to engage the gearshift in drive, the CMC joint of the thumb was adducted 5 degrees and the IP joint of the thumb was flexed 5 degrees to maintain the hold on the gearshift.

As the right upper extremity moved from the key to the gearshift, the majority of the muscular activity was concentric in nature. Initially, this included the anterior deltoid and the coracobrachialis muscles, which brought the shoulder joint into position, and the biceps brachii, brachialis, and brachioradialis muscles, which positioned the elbow joint. The supinator muscle moved the forearm into position,[19-21] while the flexors carpi ulnaris and radialis muscles moved the wrist joint, with the radialis muscle having the stronger contribution due to the radial deviation that occurred.[22] The digits were controlled by the extensors pollicis longus and brevis, digitorum communis, indicis, and digiti minimi muscles.[28] This muscular activity switched to the flexors digitorum superficialis and profundus and digiti minimi as the hand began to grasp the wheel.[23-25] The adductor pollicis and the flexor pollicis longus muscles became active concentrically as the grasp was completed.[29]

As the hand was brought into its final position, the upper and lower trapezius, serratus anterior, levator scapulae, anterior deltoid, supraspinatus, and coracobrachialis muscles worked eccentrically to position the shoulder joint. The triceps brachii and the anconeus muscles positioned the elbow joint.[19-20]

The right upper extremity was then moved from the gearshift to the wheel at a 2 o'clock position (Figure 14-5). The shoulder joint adducted 20 degrees. The elbow joint maintained its flexed position. The forearm pronated 25 degrees, bringing the forearm to 20 degrees of pronation. The wrist joint remained in flexion and radial deviation. The hand assumed a cylindrical grip on the wheel, similar to the left hand.

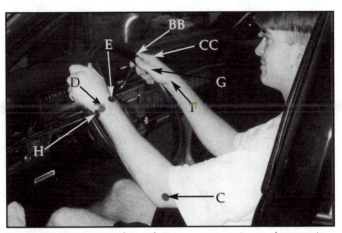

Figure 14-5. Moving the right upper extremity to the steering wheel: The subject released his cylindrical grip on the gear shift and moved the right hand to the steering wheel, resuming the use of a cylindrical grip on the wheel. The key landmarks denoted by black dots are: C = lateral epicondyle of humerus; D = ulnar head (dorsal aspect); E = radial styloid process (dorsal aspect); F = radial styloid process (radial aspect); G = first MCP joint line; H = ulnar styloid process (ulnar aspect); BB = PIP joint line; and CC = MCP joint line.

The MCP joints, from two to five, were flexed 35, 50, 62, and 75 degrees, respectively; the PIP joints were flexed 85, 90, 95, and 100 degrees, respectively; and the DIP joints were flexed 35, 45, 45, and 45 degrees, respectively. The joints of the thumb were in neutral, with the thumb resting against the steering wheel.

To move from the gearshift to the wheel, the right upper extremity demonstrated all concentric activity. The serratus anterior, upper and lower trapezius, and pectoralis major muscles, working concentrically, controlled the shoulder joint. The biceps brachii and brachialis muscles, working isometrically, controlled the elbow joint, while the pronators teres and quadratus muscles, working concentrically, controlled the forearm. The wrist flexors worked isometrically to maintain the wrist flexion and radial deviation. The motions of the digits were controlled by the flexors digitorum superficialis and profundus and digiti minimi, lumbricals, and interossei, all of which worked concentrically. The flexor pollicis brevis and adductor pollicis muscles worked concentrically to bring the thumb into its resting position on the steering wheel.[23-25,29]

Steering the Car

The left and right upper extremities maintained their positions on the steering wheel as the car picked up speed and moved forward. The muscular activities of both upper extremities were mainly isometric in nature to maintain the positions.

Slowing Down the Car

When slowing down the car, the subject maintained the upper extremity positions on the steering wheel. The motions and muscular activities previously cited continued.

Applying the Brake

When the car had been brought to a stop, the right upper extremity moved the gear shift from drive to park and then returned to the key to stop the ignition (Figure 14-6). These motions were the reverse of those cited for the initial steps of starting the ignition and moving the gearshift into drive.

PART 2: LOWER EXTREMITY ANALYSIS WITH AUTOMATIC TRANSMISSION

Starting the Engine

The subject's feet were resting on the floor as the activity began. Both ankles were plantarflexed 30 degrees at this time. The left lower extremity remained in its starting position throughout this portion of the activity. As the key was turned, the right foot was moved to the gas pedal. The right ankle joint remained in its starting position as the foot was brought to the gas pedal. Motions occurring more proximally moved the foot into position. For the remainder of the activity related to the gas pedal, the right heel remained on the floor, with motions occurring at the ankle joint to activate the gas pedal. The dorsiflexors, working isometrically, maintained the position of the right ankle during this initial movement.[30-31]

The left knee was flexed to 50 degrees, and the right knee was flexed to 95 degrees at the starting position. The right knee joint was extended 45 degrees as the right foot was positioned on the gas pedal (Figure 14-7). The quadriceps femoris muscle was active to position the right knee joint. An eccentric contraction controlled the movement of the knee to allow the placement of the foot on the pedal.[32]

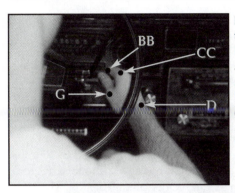

Figure 14-6. Turning off the ignition: The subject used the right hand to turn the key backward and stop the engine. A lateral prehension grip was used. The key landmarks denoted by black dots are: D = ulnar head (dorsal aspect); G = first MCP joint line; BB = PIP joint line; and CC = MCP joint line.

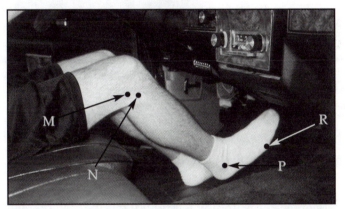

Figure 14-7. Starting the engine: The right lower extremity was moved to the gas pedal as the ignition was started. The key landmarks denoted by black dots are: M = lateral epicondyle of femur; N = fibular head; P = lateral malleolus; and R = fifth MTT joint line (lateral aspect).

In the starting position, both hips were in 86 degrees of flexion. The right hip joint moved to 92 degrees of flexion and 2 degrees of abduction. The iliopsoas and tensor fascia latae muscles worked concentrically to cause these motions.[33] The gluteus medius, a prime abductor of the hip joint, was not in a position to be most effective as an abductor during this phase due to the flexed position of the hip joint.

Accelerating the Car

During phase 2, the car was accelerated to 25 miles per hour. The right foot pressed down on the gas pedal as the right ankle joint was plantarflexed an additional 6 degrees. The plantarflexors worked concentrically to push the foot downward.[34]

During this entire phase, the knee joints maintained their positions. The quadriceps femoris muscles worked isometrically to control the position of both knee joints;[32] the same was true for the hip joints. Isometric contractions of iliopsoas and tensor fascia latae controlled the position of the right hip.[35-36] The left hip was passively positioned against the seat.

Increasing the Speed of the Car

During phase 3, in which the speed was being increased to 25 miles per hour, the right ankle joint was plantarflexed an additional 5 degrees, bringing the right ankle joint to 41 degrees of plantarflexion. The right soleus muscle worked concentrically to produce the needed motion.

The right knee joint was being extended in this phase, moving from 50 degrees of flexion to 45 degrees of flexion. The right quadriceps femoris muscle worked concentrically to produce this motion. At the same time, the right hip joint was moving from 92 degrees to 90 degrees of flexion toward extension. Concentric activity of the gluteus maximus and hamstring muscles produced this motion.

Slowing Down the Car

The next phase involved the slowing down process, in which pressure on the gas pedal was decreased. The right ankle dorsiflexed gradually, coming to rest at 25 degrees of plantarflexion. The dorsiflexor muscles worked concentrically to produce this motion. The right knee increased in flexion 5 degrees, returning to 50 degrees. This motion was produced by the concentric activity of the hamstring muscles. The right hip joint also increased in flexion, returning to its 92 degrees of flexion. The iliopsoas muscle worked concentrically to produce this motion of the hip joint. As previously stated, the left lower extremity maintained its original position.

Applying the Brake

In the final phase, the brake was applied in order to bring the car to a complete stop. The right foot moved from the gas pedal to the brake pedal to depress it (Figure 14-8), and the car came to a complete stop.

The right ankle joint began this phase in 25 degrees of plantarflexion and moved in the direction of plantarflexion and inversion. By the end of the phase, the right ankle had moved to 30 degrees of plantarflexion and 7 degrees of inversion through a concentric contraction of the soleus and posterior tibialis muscles.[30-31,34]

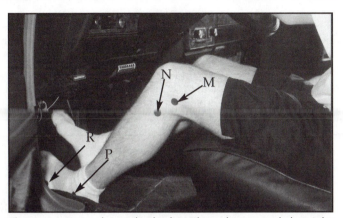

Figure 14-8. Applying the brake: The subject used the right foot to push downward on the brake and stop the car. The key landmarks denoted by black dots are: M = lateral epicondyle of femur; N = fibular head; P = malleolus; and R = fifth MTT joint line (lateral aspect).

The right knee joint decreased its flexion from 50 to 45 degrees. The quadriceps femoris produced this extension component by working concentrically.[32] Initially, the right hip joint flexed an additional 5 degrees and adducted 10 degrees to move the foot to the brake pedal. These movements were brought about by concentric activity of the iliopsoas and the adductors.[35] By the end of the phase, the right hip joint decreased in flexion, returning to 87 degrees of flexion. The gluteus maximus and hamstrings had worked concentrically to produce this final motion.

COMPARISON TO DRIVING WITH A MANUAL TRANSMISSION

Driving with a manual transmission is somewhat similar to using an automatic transmission. One obvious difference is the need for coordinated movement of both lower extremities to control the gas pedal and the clutch, while the right upper extremity works the gearshift.

The starting position for this analysis was similar to that used for the automatic transmission. One additional measurement, the distance from the seat to the clutch, was 118 inches. This was an inch shorter than the distance from the seat to the brake because the clutch protruded upward more. The ignition slot was located on the lower aspect of the dashboard facing the driver. It was 5 inches from the gearshift. All other measurements were the same.

The first part of this comparison focused on the activities of the upper extremities and was divided into several phases for ease of understanding: phase 1 covered the starting position to starting the engine; phase 2 covered moving from one gear to another; phase 3 covered steering the car; phase 4 covered slowing down the car; and phase 5 covered applying the brake.

The second part of this analysis focused on the activities of the lower extremities and was divided into similar phases: phase 1 covered starting the engine; phase 2, accelerating the car; phase 3, shifting from first to second gear; phase 4, shifting from second to third gear; and phase 5, increasing the speed. Three additional phases were needed to cover the activities of the lower extremities: phase 6 covered slowing down the car; phase 7, releasing the clutch; and phase 8, applying the brake.

PART 1: UPPER EXTREMITY ANALYSIS WITH MANUAL TRANSMISSION

Starting the Engine

Beginning in the established starting position, the right upper extremity was in 45 degrees of shoulder forward flexion and 10 degrees of abduction. The elbow joint was flexed 45 degrees, and the forearm was pronated 70 degrees. The wrist joint was extended 30 degrees and radially deviated 15 degrees. The hand was using a lateral prehension-type grip to grasp the key.[16] The CMC joint of the thumb was flexed 8 degrees; the MCP joint, 34 degrees; and the IP joint was in neutral. The MCP joints of digits two through five were flexed 52, 70, 70, and 66 degrees, respectively. The PIP joints were flexed 20, 15, 10, and 8 degrees, respectively. The DIP joints of digits two through four were flexed 5, 4, and 1 degrees, respectively. The DIP joint of the fifth digit was in neutral.

As the key was turned halfway to the right, the shoulder joint maintained its original position. The elbow joint flexed an additional 5 degrees, and the forearm was supinated 30 degrees, bringing the forearm to 40 degrees of pronation. The wrist joint was flexed 65 degrees, bringing it to 35 degrees of flexion. The wrist joint was also ulnarly deviated 35 degrees, bringing it to 20 degrees of ulnar deviation. The positions of the digits remained the same.

From a muscular perspective, there was an interplay between isometric activity and concentric activity to operate the car. In the initial key turning aspect, the right shoulder muscles (upper and lower trapezius, serratus anterior, levator scapulae, anterior deltoid, supraspinatus, and coracobrachialis) worked isometrically to maintain the shoulder position.[17-18]

The biceps brachii, brachialis, and brachioradialis worked concentrically to control the elbow motion. The supinator and biceps brachii muscles worked concentrically to control the forearm position.[19-21] The flexors carpi ulnaris and radialis muscles worked concentrically at the wrist joint, with the flexor carpi ulnaris having the greater contribution due to the ulnar deviation needed at this time.[22] The muscles of the digits (flexors pollicis longus and brevis, flexors digitorum superficialis and profundus, flexor digit minimi, lumbricals, and interossei) all worked isometrically to maintain the grasp on the key.

To start the ignition, the key was turned completely to the right. Once again, the shoulder joint maintained its original position. The elbow joint extended 5 degrees, bringing the elbow joint to 45 degrees of flexion. The forearm was supinated an additional 5 degrees, bringing the forearm to 35 degrees of pronation. The wrist joint was flexed an additional 3 degrees, bringing it to 38 degrees of flexion. The wrist joint was ulnarly deviated an additional 5 degrees, bringing it to 25 degrees of ulnar deviation. The position of the digits had not changed.

To complete the turning of the key, the shoulder musculature continued its isometric work. The triceps brachii and anconeus muscles worked concentrically to extend the elbow.[26-27] The supinator and biceps brachii muscles continued to work concentrically to supinate the forearm. The wrist flexors also continued their concentric activity, with the flexor carpi ulnaris muscle contributing more to the activity due to the continuing ulnar deviation. The muscles of the digits continued isometrically to maintain the grasp on the key.

During this entire procedure, the left upper extremity remained in position on the steering wheel. The shoulder joint was in 50 degrees of flexion; the elbow joint, in 105 degrees of flexion; the forearm, in 45 degrees of pronation; and the wrist joint, in 25 degrees of ulnar deviation. The hand maintained a cylindrical grip on the wheel. All the joints of digits two through five were in varying degrees of flexion. The MCP joints, from two to five, were flexed 35, 50, 62, and 75 degrees, respectively; the PIP joints were flexed 60, 75, 75, and 55 degrees, respectively; and the DIP joints were flexed 35, 45, 30, and 17 degrees, respectively. The thumb was held in neutral, resting against the wheel.

During this entire time, the muscles of the left upper extremity worked isometrically to maintain the position of the left upper extremity on the wheel. The upper and lower trapezius, serratus anterior, latissimus dorsi, anterior deltoid, supraspinatus, and coracobrachialis muscles were active at the shoulder joint.[17-18] The biceps brachii and brachialis muscles were active at the elbow joint. The pronators teres and quadratus muscles controlled the forearm position.[19-21] The flexor carpi ulnaris and the extensor carpi ulnaris muscles controlled the wrist position.[22] The flexor digitorum profundus muscle maintained the position of the digits.[23-25]

Moving the Right Upper Extremity to the Gearshift

Once the ignition was started, the right upper extremity moved from the key to the gearshift to engage it in the first drive position. The shoulder joint extended 25 degrees, while the elbow joint flexed 25 degrees and the forearm pronated 45 degrees. The joints of all the digits extended 25 degrees to release the grip on the key and then flexed 30 degrees to grasp the gearshift. However, the thumb remained in the extended position as it was brought around the gearshift. As the shoulder and elbow joints extended an additional 5 degrees each to engage the gearshift in drive, the CMC joint adducted 5 degrees and its IP joint flexed 5 degrees to maintain its opposition to the gearshift.

As the right upper extremity moved from the key to the gearshift, the majority of the muscular activity was concentric in nature. Initially, this included the middle trapezius, rhomboids major and minor, latissimus dorsi, and posterior deltoid muscles, which brought the shoulder joint into position, and the biceps brachii, brachialis, and brachioradialis muscles, which positioned the elbow joint. The pronators teres and quadratus muscles moved the forearm into position,[19-21] while the flexors carpi ulnaris and radialis muscles moved the wrist joint. There was a continued greater contribution from the flexor carpi ulnaris due to the continued ulnar deviation.[22] The digits were controlled by the extensors pollicis longus and brevis, digitorum communis, indicis, and digiti minimi muscles.[28] This muscular activity switched to the flexors digitorum superficialis and profundus and digiti minimi as the hand began to grasp the wheel.[23-25] The adductor pollicis and the flexor pollicis longus muscles became active concentrically as the grasp was completed.[29]

As the hand was brought into its final position, the upper and lower trapezius, serratus anterior, levator scapulae, anterior deltoid, supraspinatus, and coracobrachialis muscles worked concentrically to position the shoulder joint. The triceps brachii and the anconeus muscles positioned the elbow joint.[19-20]

The right upper extremity was then moved from the gearshift to the wheel at a 2 o'clock position. The shoulder joint flexed 30 degrees and adducted 35 degrees. The elbow joint flexed 45 degrees, and the forearm supinated 60 degrees. The wrist joint flexed 10 degrees and ulnarly deviated 35 degrees. The hand assumed a cylindrical grip on the wheel, similar to the left hand. The MCP joints, from two to five, were flexed 35, 50, 62, and 75 degrees, respectively; the PIP joints were flexed 60, 75, 75, and 55 degrees, respectively; and the DIP joints were flexed 35, 45,

30, and 17 degrees, respectively. The CMC joint of the thumb was flexed 10 degrees and adducted 5 degrees.

To move from the gearshift to the wheel, the right upper extremity demonstrated all concentric activity. The serratus anterior, upper and lower trapezius, pectoralis major, anterior deltoid, and coracobrachialis muscles controlled the shoulder joint. The biceps brachii, brachialis, and brachioradialis muscles controlled the elbow joint, while the supinator and biceps brachii controlled the forearm. The flexors carpi ulnaris and radialis muscles moved the wrist into position, with the flexor carpi ulnaris giving a greater contribution due to the ulnar deviation of the wrist at this time. The motions of the digits were controlled by the flexors digitorum superficialis and profundus and digiti minimi, lumbricals, interossei, flexor pollicis brevis, and adductor pollicis muscles.[23-25,29]

Moving from One Gear to Another

The process described above was repeated as the car gained speed, and the gearshift was moved from first to second to third gear. The right upper extremity alternated positions from the wheel to the gearshift and back again. The pattern of muscular activity described above continued as the subject switched from one gear to another.

Steering the Car

The left upper extremity maintained its position on the steering wheel as the car picked up speed and moved forward. The right upper extremity moved back and forth between the steering wheel and the gearshift until sufficient speed had been reached. The motions and muscular activities of both upper extremities were the same as those previously cited.

Slowing Down the Car (Downshifting to Second Gear)

To slow down the car, the subject again shifted the right upper extremity back and forth between the steering wheel and the gearshift, this time moving from third to second gear and then from second to first gear. The left upper extremity maintained its position on the wheel. The previously cited motions and muscular activities continued.

Applying the Brake

When the car had been brought to a stop, the right upper extremity pushed the gearshift upward to put it in park and then returned to the key to its start position to stop the engine. These motions were the reverse of those cited for the initial steps of starting the ignition and putting the gearshift into first gear.

PART 2: LOWER EXTREMITY ANALYSIS WITH MANUAL TRANSMISSION

Starting the Engine

The subject's feet were resting on the floor. By midposition, the left foot was resting on the clutch, and the right foot had depressed the gas pedal. By the end of this phase, the left foot had depressed the clutch, and the right foot was resting on the gas pedal. Both ankle joints were plantarflexed 30 degrees as this activity began. The left ankle joint dorsiflexed 28 degrees as it was brought to rest on the clutch. The dorsiflexors, working concentrically, achieved this motion.[30-31] By the end of this phase, the left ankle was plantarflexed 33 degrees. The plantarflexors worked concentrically as the clutch was depressed. The soleus component was the primary mover during this time due to the flexed position of the knee joint.[30,34] The right ankle joint remained in its starting position as it was brought to the gas pedal through motions occurring more proximally. For the remainder of the activity related to the gas pedal, the right heel remained on the floor, with motions occurring at the ankle joint to activate the gas pedal. The dorsiflexors, working isometrically, maintained the position of the right ankle.

The knee joints were flexed to 95 degrees at the starting position. The left knee moved to 74 degrees of flexion as the left foot was moved to the clutch. As the clutch was depressed, the left knee moved to 27 degrees of flexion. The quadriceps femoris muscle worked concentrically to bring about the extension movements of this phase.[32]

The right knee was extended 55 degrees as the right foot was positioned on the gas pedal. From this position of 40 degrees of flexion, the right knee joint moved to 65 degrees of flexion as the right foot came to rest on the gas pedal. In both instances, the quadriceps femoris muscle was active. Initially, this muscle worked concentrically. However, as the movement continued, the contraction reversed to eccentric to control the placement of the foot on the pedal.[32]

In the starting position, both hip joints were in 86 degrees of flexion. The flexion of the left hip joint increased to 92 degrees as the left foot was brought to rest on the clutch. The iliopsoas was used concentrically to achieve this position. At the same time, the left hip adducted 7 degrees, having been moved by a concentric contraction of the hip adductors. By the end of this phase, the left hip had extended 26 degrees to position the foot on the clutch. To bring the hip into this 66 degrees of flexion, the iliopsoas reversed its contraction to eccentric.

This eccentric activity of the iliopsoas muscle provided the control needed on the clutch. The left hip was abducted 7 degrees by a concentric contraction of the tensor fascia latae.[36] The gluteus medius muscle, normally the prime abductor of the hip joint, was not in a position to be most effective as an abductor due to the flexed position of the hip joint.

The right hip joint moved to 74 degrees of flexion and 2 degrees of abduction. The iliopsoas worked eccentrically, while the tensor fascia latae worked concentrically to cause these motions. By the end of this phase, the right hip flexed an additional 4 degrees to position the right foot on the pedal. The iliopsoas muscle reversed its activity to concentric to complete this motion. This reversal of lower extremity muscle activity was seen to continue throughout this phase, as there was need for control of the motions occurring to successfully manipulate the clutch and the gas pedal.

Accelerating the Car

During this phase, the car was accelerated from 0 to 10 miles per hour. During this time, the transmission had been put into first gear. The left foot eased up on the clutch so that it was depressed halfway, while the right foot pressed down on the gas pedal so that it was depressed halfway. By the end of this phase, the left foot was resting on the clutch once again, and the right foot further depressed the gas pedal to increase the speed to 15 miles per hour.

As this phase began, the left ankle moved into 18 degrees of plantarflexion to resist the upward force of the clutch. The plantarflexors worked eccentrically to control this motion. By the end of this phase, plantarflexion had been decreased further to 2 degrees, with the plantarflexors continuing their eccentric activity. The right ankle moved from 3 to 6 degrees of plantarflexion as pressure was exerted downward on the gas pedal. The plantarflexors worked concentrically to push the foot downward. By the end of this phase, another 3 degrees of plantarflexion had occurred through continued concentric contractions of the plantarflexors.[34]

Initially, the left knee joint was flexed another 23 degrees and, by the end of this phase, was flexed another 24 degrees to end in 74 degrees of flexion. The quadriceps femoris muscle worked eccentrically to control these motions of the left knee. The right knee joint decreased its flexion range from 65 to 62 degrees at the start of this phase. By the end of this phase, the flexion had decreased an additional 3 degrees, ending at 59 degrees. On this side, the quadriceps femoris muscle worked similarly to control the right knee joint.[32]

The left hip joint was flexing from 66 to 92 degrees in response to the force generated by the clutch. Eccentric activity of the gluteus maximus and hamstring muscles worked to control the amount of hip flexion. The right hip joint was extending from 8 to 74 degrees of flexion. Concentric contractions of the gluteus maximus and hamstring muscles worked to push the lower extremity downward on the gas pedal.[35-36]

Shifting From First to Second Gear

In this phase, the subject shifted the transmission from first to second gear. The left foot pressed halfway down on the clutch, while the right foot eased up on the gas pedal, releasing it halfway. By the end of this phase, the clutch had been depressed, and the right foot was resting on the gas pedal.

Beginning at 2 degrees of plantarflexion, the left ankle joint moved to 35 degrees of plantarflexion. The soleus worked concentrically the entire time to bring about this plantarflexion.[34] The right ankle moved from 9 to 3 degrees of plantarflexion. The dorsiflexors worked concentrically throughout this phase.[31]

The left knee joint started at 74 degrees of flexion and moved to 27 degrees of flexion. The quadriceps femoris muscle brought about this extension motion by working concentrically. The right knee joint increased in flexion from 59 to 65 degrees throughout this phase. The hamstring muscles worked concentrically to cause the flexion.

During this phase, the left hip joint decreased it flexion from 92 to 66 degrees. Concentric activity of the gluteus maximus muscle helped to depress the clutch during this phase. The right hip joint had increased in flexion from 74 to 78 degrees. The gluteus maximus worked eccentrically to control the movements of the right hip.[35-36]

Speed was increased from 10 to 20 miles per hour in this phase. Once again, the left foot eased up on the clutch, releasing it halfway, while the right foot pressed down on the gas pedal. The left foot rested on the clutch, while the right foot maintained pressure on the gas pedal to accelerate the car to 20 miles per hour.

The left ankle joint motion was a reversal of that seen in the previous phase. The soleus muscle worked eccentrically to resist the upward force of the clutch. The motion of the right ankle joint was a gradual increase in plantarflexion, moving from 3 to 14 degrees of plantarflexion throughout this phase. The soleus acted concentrically to produce this motion on the right side.

The left knee and hip joint motions and muscular activities were the same as those seen in the second phase. The right knee, through concentric work of the quadriceps femoris muscle, moved from 65 to 51 degrees of flexion. The right hip joint moved from 78 to 71 degrees of flexion. This motion was brought about by concentric contractions of the hamstring and gluteus maximus muscles.

Shifting From Second to Third Gear

Phase 5 was a repeat of phase 3, with the transmission being shifted from second to third gear. The left ankle began this phase in 2 degrees of plantarflexion and, by the end of the phase, moved to 35 degrees of plantarflexion. The soleus worked concentrically during this entire time. The right ankle decreased its plantarflexion during this phase, moving from 14 to 3 degrees of plantarflexion, through concentric activity of the dorsiflexors.

The left knee joint was extended from 74 to 27 degrees of flexion by the quadriceps femoris acting concentrically. The right knee joint, moved by the concentric contractions of the hamstring muscles, was flexed from 51 to 65 degrees throughout this phase.

The left hip joint motion and muscular activity was a repeat of that seen in phase 3. The right hip moved into greater flexion throughout this phase. Motion started at 71 degrees and moved to 78 degrees of flexion. The iliopsoas muscle contracted concentrically to produce the increased flexion.

Increasing the Speed of the Car

Phase 6 was a repeat of phase 4, with the speed being increased to 25 miles per hour. The left ankle joint, controlled by eccentric contractions of the soleus muscle, was dorsiflexed from 35 to 2 degrees of plantarflexion. The right ankle joint was plantarflexed during this time, moving from 3 to 20 degrees of plantarflexion. The right soleus muscle worked concentrically to produce the needed motion.

The left knee joint increased in flexion from 27 to 74 degrees. Eccentric activity of the quadriceps femoris muscle controlled this motion. The right knee joint, moving from 65 to 44 degrees of flexion, was extended in this phase. The right quadriceps femoris worked concentrically to produce this motion.

The left hip joint was flexed from 66 to 92 degrees during this time. Motion was brought about by eccentric activity of the gluteus maximus and hamstring muscles to control the force produced by the clutch. The right hip joint was moving from 78 to 68 degrees of flexion toward extension. Concentric activity of the gluteus maximus and hamstring muscles produced this extension.

Slowing Down the Car

The next phase involved the slowing down process, in which the transmission was downshifted from third to second gear. Again, this phase was similar to phase 5. The motions and the muscular activities of the joints on the left side were the same as those seen in phase 5.

The motions on the right side varied from those seen in phase 5 but followed a similar pattern. The right ankle moved from 20 to 3 degrees of plantarflexion, being moved by the concentric contraction of the dorsiflexors. Flexion of the right knee, produced by the concentric activity of the hamstring muscles, increased from 44 to 65 degrees. The right hip joint increased in flexion from 68 to 78 degrees, produced by the iliopsoas muscle working concentrically.

Releasing the Clutch

Phase 8 involved releasing the clutch to slow down the car. In this phase, the left foot released the clutch halfway, while the right foot remained resting on the gas pedal, which had been released halfway during the preceding phase.

The left ankle reversed the motion seen in the previous phase, which decreased the amount of plantarflexion. The soleus worked eccentrically to resist the upward force of the clutch. The left knee joint also reversed the motion seen in the previous phase, thereby increasing its flexion. The quadriceps femoris muscle worked eccentrically to control the force of the clutch. The right lower extremity remained in the same position assumed at the end of the last phase. Isometric muscle contractions maintained the position of the right lower extremity.

Applying the Brake

In the final phase, the brake was applied to bring the car to a complete stop. The left foot depressed the clutch, while the right foot moved from the gas to the brake pedal. By the end of this phase, the right foot had depressed the brake pedal, and the car had come to a complete stop.

The left ankle joint began this phase in 2 degrees of plantarflexion and moved into more plantarflexion as the phase continued. By the end of this phase, the left ankle joint was in 35 degrees of plantarflexion, with motion produced by the concentric contraction of the soleus muscle. The right ankle joint began this phase in 3 degrees of plantarflexion and moved in the direction of dorsiflexion and inversion. By midphase, the right ankle joint was dorsiflexed 13 degrees and inverted 9 degrees. Both motions were produced by the tibialis anterior muscle working concentrically. By the end of the phase, the right ankle had moved to 8 degrees of plantarflexion through a concentric contraction of the soleus muscle.[30-31,34]

The left knee joint decreased its flexion from 74 to 27 degrees during this phase. The quadriceps femoris muscle was working concentrically to produce the flexion. The right knee joint increased its flexion from 65 to 67 degrees by midphase. The hamstrings, working concentrically, produced this motion. By the end of this phase, the right knee joint had moved to 61 degrees of flexion. The quadriceps femoris produced this extension component by working concentrically.[32]

The left hip joint decreased its flexion from 92 to 66 degrees. The gluteus maximus and hamstrings worked concentrically at the left hip.[35-36] The right hip joint increased its flexion from 78 to 83 degrees by midphase. In addition, the right hip adducted 5 degrees. These movements were brought about by concentric activity of the iliopsoas and the adductors. By the end of the phase, the right hip joint was in 75 degrees of flexion. The gluteus maximus and hamstrings had worked concentrically to produce this final motion.

For those individuals who drive a manual transmission, the activity of the lower extremities was different. The left lower extremity was used to control the pedals. In addition, there was more activity of the upper extremities as the gearshift was moved from one gear to another. Range of motions varied considerably in these two analyses. These differences were due to the variations in how each type of transmission worked.

SUMMARY

Key Anatomical Landmarks for Driving Analysis

Upper Extremity Components

Shoulder Complex: Greater tuberosity of humerus
Acromion process (superior aspect)

Elbow and Forearm   Lateral epicondyle of humerus
Complex: Radial styloid process (dorsal aspect)
Radial styloid process (lateral aspect)
Ulnar head (dorsal aspect)
Ulnar styloid process (ulnar aspect)

Wrist and Hand   Base of first MCP (radial and palmar aspects)
Complex: Base of second MCP (dorsal aspect)
Base of fifth MCP (dorsal aspect)

First MCP joint line (palmar aspect)
Second MCP joint line (radial aspect)
Fifth MCP joint line (ulnar aspect)
First IP joint line (palmar aspect)
Second PIP joint line (radial aspect)
Fifth PIP joint line (ulnar aspect)
Second DIP joint line (radial aspect)
Fifth DIP joint line (ulnar aspect)

Lower Extremity Components

Hip Complex: Greater trochanter of femur

Knee Complex: Lateral epicondyle of femur
                      Medial epicondyle of femur
                      Fibular head

Ankle and Foot   Lateral malleolus
Complex: Medial malleolus
                      Fifth MTP joint line (lateral aspect)

Major Phases for Driving Analysis

Starting Position

- Position of subject
- Position of seat

Upper Extremity Analysis

- Starting the engine
- Moving the right upper extremity to the gearshift
- Steering the car
- Slowing down the car
- Applying the brake

Lower Extremity Analysis

- Starting the engine
- Accelerating the car
- Increasing the speed of the car
- Slowing down the car
- Applying the brake

Joint Motions and Muscular Activity: Driving a Car

Introduction and Set-Up: Right Upper Extremity

• Primarily flexion of proximal and distal joints.

• Pronation of radioulnar joint and radial deviation of wrist joint.

Starting the Engine: Right Upper Extremity

• Initially, primarily flexion of elbow and wrist joints.

• Supination of radioulnar joint followed by extension of elbow joint.

• Primarily concentric muscular contractions.

Starting the Engine: Left Upper Extremity

• Primarily fixed flexion of proximal and distal joints via isometric muscular activity.

Moving the Right Upper Extremity to the Gearshift

• Primarily flexion of proximal joints.

• Extension, followed by flexion of digits.

• Concentric contractions of all muscles.

Steering and Slowing Down the Car

• Both upper extremities maintained their positions via isometric muscular contractions.

Applying the Brake

• Motions are the reverse of those cited for the initial step of starting the ignition and moving the gearshift into drive.

Introduction and Set-Up: Lower Extremities

• All proximal joints are flexed.

• Ankle joints are plantarflexed.

Starting the Engine

• Flexion and abduction of right hip.

• Extension of right knee.

• All concentric muscular contractions.

Accelerating the Car

• Primarily plantarflexion of right ankle joint via concentric muscular activity.

Increasing the Speed of the Car

• Extension of proximal joints.

• Plantarflexion of right ankle joint.

• All concentric muscular contractions.

Slowing Down the Car

• Flexion of all joints via concentric muscular contractions.

Applying the Brake

• Flexion, followed by extension of right hip joint.

• Extension of right knee joint.

• Plantarflexion and inversion of right ankle joint.

• All concentric muscular contractions.

Differences Between Automatic Transmission and Manual Transmission Usage

• The major difference in usage involved the need for the left lower extremity to control the pedals in addition to the right lower extremity.

• There was more right upper extremity usage as the right upper extremity moved from one gear to another.

CLINICAL APPLICATION AND DISCUSSION QUESTIONS

No lower extremity activity would be needed for those individuals who use hand controls. What is the role of the upper extremities in such a car? Compare upper extremity usage to those cited in the two analyses in this chapter.

Think about the interior design of different types of automobiles. How may the interior design affect the analysis of the extremities?

Although the spinal components were not covered in this analysis, think about these. Are all areas of the spine involved in the activity? How important are the cervical components in operating a vehicle? How would low back pain affect the manner in which an individual drives?

Think about the biomechanics of entering and exiting a car. Compare a four-door car to a two-door car. How does this differ from entering and exiting a truck?

Do an analysis of driving a motorcycle. How does it compare to that of driving a car? Next, analyze mounting a motorcycle. How does it compare to mounting a bicycle?

Finally, generate a list of muscle substitutions. Compare your substitutions to Charts 1 and 2 in Appendix A.

REFERENCES

1. Ayoub MM. Sitting down on the job (properly). *Industrial Design.* 1972;19:42-45.
2. Roberts DF. Passenger comfort-seating. *Bus and Coach.* 1963;35:214-219.
3. Thier RH. Measurement of seat comfort. *Automotive Engineering.* 1963;53:64-66.

4. Jacobs H, Sussman D, Abernathy C, Plank G, Stoklosa J. Please remain seated: seat designs to help retain passengers during emergency stops. Proceedings of the Human Factors Society 24th Annual Meeting. 1980.

5. Severy DM, Brink HM, Baird JD. Rigid seats with 28 inch seatback effectively reduce injuries in 30+ mph rear-end impacts. *Society of Automotive Engineers Journal*. 1969;77:20-25.

6. LeCapentier EF. Easy chair dimension for comfort—a subjective approach. Proceedings of the Symposium on Sitting Posture. 1969.

7. Oxford HW. Factors in the design of seats used in public transport. Proceedings of the Tenth Annual Conference of the Ergonomics Society of Australia and New Zealand. 1973.

8. Corlett EN, Eklund JAE. How does a backrest work? *Appl Ergonomics*. 1984;15:111-114.

9. Floyd WF. Postural factors in the design of motor car seats. Proceedings of the Royal Society of Medicine. 1967;60:953-955.

10. Hall EC. Seating for transportation. Proceedings of the 20th Annual Conference of the Ergonomics Society of Australia and New Zealand. 1983.

11. Hartnett B. Is the modern motor car ergonomically efficient? Proceedings of the 17th Annual Conference of the Ergonomics Society of Australia and New Zealand. 1980.

12. Radke AO. *The Importance of Seating in Driver Comfort and Performance*.Detroit, Mich: Society of Automotive Engineers, publication no. 838B; 1964.

13. Rebiffé R. An ergonomic study of the arrangement of the driving position in motor cars. *Proceedings of the Institution of Mechanical Engineers*. 1966;181(part 3D):43-50.

14. Varterasian JH, Thompson RR. *The Dynamic Characteristics of Automobile Seats with Human Occupants*. Detroit, Mich: Society of Automotive Engineers, publication no. 770249; 1977.

15. Department of Law and Public Safety; Division of Motor Vehicles. *New Jersey Driver Manual*. Trenton, NJ: New Jersey Department of Transportation;94.

16. Landsmeer JMF. Power grip and precision handling. *Ann Rheum Dis*. 1962;21:164-170.

17. DeLuca CJ, Forrest WJ. Force analysis of individual muscles acting simultaneously on the shoulder joint during isometric abduction. *J Biomech*. 1973;6:385-393.

18. Kronberg M, Nemeth G, Brostrom L. Muscle activity and coordination in the normal shoulder. *Clin Orthop*. 1990;257:76-85.

19. Basmajian JV, Latif A. Integrated actions and functions of the chief flexors of the elbow: a detailed electromyographic analysis. *J Bone Joint Surg Am*. 1957;39:1106-1118.

20. Pauly JE, Rushing JL, Scheving LE. An electromyographic study of some muscles crossing the elbow joint. *Anat Rec.* 1967;159:47-53.

21. Ray RD, Johnson RJ, Jameson RM. Rotation of the forearm: an experimental study of pronation and supination. *J Bone Joint Surg Am.* 1951;33;993-996.

22. Kauer JMG. Functional anatomy of the wrist. *Clin Orthop.* 1980;149:9-20.

23. An KN, Chao EY, Cooney WP, Linscheid RI. Normative model of human hand for biomechanical analysis. *J Biomech.* 1979;12:775-788.

24. Chao EY, Opgrande JR, Axmear FE. Three-dimensional force analysis of finger joints in selected isometric hand functions. *J Biomech.* 1976;9:387-396.

25. Long C, Conrad PW, Hall EA, Furler SL. Intrinsic-extrinsic muscle control of the hand in power grip and precision handling: an electromyographic study. *J Bone Joint Surg Br.* 1970;52:853-867.

26. Little AD, Lehmkuhl D. Elbow extension force measured in three positions. *Phys Ther.* 1966;46:7-17.

27. Basmajian JV, Griffin WR. Function of anconeus muscle: an electromyographic study. *J Bone Joint Surg Am.* 1972;54:1712-1714.

28. Sunderland S. Actions of the extensor digitorum communis, interosseous, and lumbrical muscles. *American Journal of Anatomy.* 1945;77:189-194.

29. Iameda T, An K, Cooney WP. Functional anatomy and biomechanics of the thumb. *Hand Clin.* 1992;8:9-15.

30. DiStefano V. Anatomy and biomechanics of the ankle and foot. *Athletic Training.* 1981;16:43-47.

31. Ambagtsheer JBT. The function of the muscles of the lower leg in relation to movements of the tarsus. *Acta Orthop Scand.* 1978;172(suppl):1-196.

32. Duarte-Cintra AI, Furlani J. Electromyographic study of quadriceps femoris in man. *Electromyogr Clin Neurophysiol.* 1981;21:539-554.

33. Pare EB, Stern JT, Schwartz JM. Functional differentiation within the tensor fasciae latae. *J Bone Joint Surg Am.* 1981;63:1457-1471.

34. Furlani J, Vitti M, Costacurta L. Electromyographic behavior of the gastrocnemius muscle. *Electromyogr Clin Neurophysiol.* 1978;18:29-34.

35. Dostal WF, Andrews JG. A three-dimensional biomechanical model of hip musculature. *J Biomech.* 1981;14:803-812.

36. Nemeth G, Ekholm J, Arborelius UP, et al. Influence of knee flexion on isometric hip extensor strength. *Scand J Rehabil Med.* 1983;15:97-101.

SUGGESTED READINGS

Andersson GBJ, Ortengren R, Nachemson A, Elfström G. Lumbar disc pressure and myoelectric back muscle activity during sitting. *Scand J Rehab Med.* 1974;6(part 4):128-133.

Bean LE. Car transfer technique of a patient with quadriplegia. *Phys Ther.* 1969;49:602-604.

Bogduk N. The anatomy and pathophysiology of whiplash. *Clin Biomech.* 1986;1:92-101.

Brand RA, Crowninshield RD, Johnston RC, Pedersen DR. Forces on the femoral head during activities of daily living. *Iowa Orthop J.* 1982;2:43-49.

Clark MC, Faletti MV. The role of seating types in egress difficulty experienced by older adults: a biomechanical analysis. In: RW Swezey, ed. *Proceedings of the Human Factors Society 29th Annual Meeting.* Baltimore, Md: 1985;343-346.

Diebschlag W, Müller-Limmroth W. Physiological requirements on car seats: some results of experimental studies. In: DJ Oborne, JA Levis, eds. *Human Factors in Transport Research.* Vol. 2. London, England: Academic Press;1980:223-230.

Hedbert G, Björkstén M, Ouchterlony-Johnsson E, Jonsson B. Rheumatic complaints among Swedish engine drivers in relation to the dimensions of the driver's cab in the Rc engine. *Appl Ergonomics.* 1981;12:93-97.

Hiba JC. Some ergonomic aspects in the design of a headrest for a passenger seat for coaches. In: DJ Oborne , JA Levis, eds. *Human Factors in Transport Research.* Vol. 2. London, England: Academic Press;1980:257-265.

Hofkosh JM, Sipajlo J, Brody L. Driver education for the physically disabled—evaluation, selection, and training methods. *Med Clin North Am.* 1969;53:685-689.

Hosea TM, Simon SR, Delatizky J, Wong MA, Hsieh CC. Myoelectric analysis of the paraspinal musculature in relation to automobile driving. *Spine.* 1986;11:928-936.

Institute for Consumer Ergonomics (ICE). *Problems Experienced by Disabled and Elderly People Entering and Leaving Cars. TRRL Research Report RR2.* Crowthorne, UK: Transport and Road Research Laboratory;1985.

Kelsey JL, Hardy EJ. Driving of motor vehicles as a risk factor for acute herniated lumbar intervertebral disc. *Am J Epidemiol.* 1975;102:63-73.

Kewman DG, Seigerman C, Kintner H, Chu S, Hensan D, Reeder C. Simulation training of psychomotor skills: teaching the brain injured to drive. *Rehabilitation Psychology.* 1985;30:11-27.

Laubenthal KN, Smidt GL, Kettelkamp DB. A quantitative analysis of knee motion during activities of daily living. *Phys Ther.* 1972;52:34-42.

Lunnen YD, Yack J, LeVeau BF. Relationship between muscle length, muscle activity, and torque of the hamstring muscles. *Phys Ther.* 1981;61:190-195.

Mayyasi AM, Pulley PE, Hyman WA, Swarts AE. Categorization of disabilities and functional limitations imposed in the driving task. *SAE Paper 730466.* SAE Automobile Engineering Meeting. Detroit, Mich. 1973.

Smidt GL. Biomechanical analysis of knee flexion and extension. *J Biomech.* 1973;6:79-92.

Troup JDG. Driver's back pain and its prevention. *Appl Ergonomics.* 1978;9:207-214.

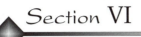

Section VI

Total Body Analysis

Chapter 15

Propelling a Wheelchair

INTRODUCTION AND SET-UP

Wheelchair propulsion varies with the type of wheelchair used by an individual. This includes design (which covers the type of backrest and seat), the diameter of the wheelbase, and the alignment of the wheels. Propulsion of a racing or sports chair is different from a regular wheelchair due to these design differences. For example, the wheels of a regular chair are aligned vertically, and the wheelbase is narrow. The force applied to the hand rim is vertical. In contrast, the wheels slant medially on a racing chair, and the wheelbase is wider. The force applied to the hand rim is diagonal and more efficient.[1-15]

This particular analysis focused on an individual who was using a standard wheelchair with sling back and seat, standard arm rests, and nonelevating leg rests. The wheelchair was 40 inches in height (measuring from the floor to the top of the handle grips), with the seat measuring 20 inches from the floor; the footrest, 6 inches from the floor; and the armrest, 30 inches from the floor. The footrest was at a 90-degree angle to the leg rest. The leg rest was set at a 34-degree angle to the wheelchair. The left armrest was removed from the wheelchair during the analysis to provide an unobstructed view of the motions of the body. The extremity analysis was limited to one side, as the opposite side mirrors the activity.

In the starting position, the subject was seated in the wheelchair with the forearms pronated and resting on the lap. From this position, the analysis looked at the activity of the subject as he leaned forward and reached backward with his upper extremities to grasp the hand rims on either side of the wheelchair. The analysis concluded with the subject propelling the wheelchair forward by bringing the upper extremities forward and then downward to turn the wheels in a counter clockwise position as one views the wheelchair from the subject's left side.

Figure 15-1. Starting position: The subject is seated upright in the wheelchair with the forearms and hands resting on the lap. The key landmarks denoted by black dots are: A = acromion process; B = greater tuberosity of humerus; C = lateral epicondyle of humerus; F = radial styloid process (radial aspect); G = first MCP joint line; J = olecranon process; M = lateral epicondyle of femur; N = fibular head; P = lateral malleolus; R = fifth MTT joint line (lateral aspect); V = greater trochanter of femur; and W = spinous process of C-7.

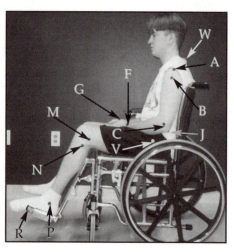

To continue propelling the wheelchair, the subject repeated the same maneuver over and over again.

With the subject seated in a relaxed position in the wheelchair (Figure 15-1), the trunk was in neutral with a slight deviation from the normal cervical lordosis due to the forward position of the subject's head. The shoulder joint was in 25 degrees of medial rotation. The elbow joint was flexed 60 degrees, and the forearm was pronated 86 degrees. The wrist joint was in 5 degrees of flexion.

The thumb CMC joint was abducted 8 degrees; the MCP joint, flexed 30 degrees; and the IP joint, flexed 35 degrees. The MCP joints of the second through fifth digits were flexed 23, 18, 12, and 10 degrees, respectively. The PIP joints were flexed 22, 20, 2, and 10 degrees, respectively. The DIP joints were in neutral. The position of the digits allowed the forearm and hand to contour to the subject's thigh as the forearm and hand rested on the subject's lap. The hip joint was flexed to 90 degrees and internally rotated 5 to 10 degrees, the knee joint was flexed to 80 degrees, and the ankle joint was in neutral.[16-24]

In this activity, muscular contraction was seen in the spinal and upper and lower extremity musculature. In the starting position (upright sitting in the wheelchair), the erector spinae muscles worked isometrically to control the posture, as did the upper trapezius, sternocleidomastoid, pectoralis major, and scalene muscles.[2-3,6-7,13,25-27]

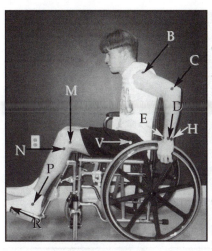

Figure 15-2. Reaching for the hand rims: The subject extended the shoulder joint to reach backwards for the hand rims. The trunk was brought forward by flexion of the hip joints. The key landmarks denoted by black dots are. B = greater tuberosity of humerus; C = lateral epicondyle of humerus; D = ulnar head (dorsal aspect); E = radial styloid process (dorsal aspect); H = ulnar styloid process (ulnar aspect); M = lateral epicondyle of femur; N = fibular head; P = lateral malleolus; R = fifth MTT joint line (lateral aspect); and V = greater trochanter of femur.

REACHING FOR THE HAND RIMS

As the subject began to reach for the hand rims (Figure 15-2), the neck was extended 15 degrees to allow the subject to keep the forward line of progression in sight. The hip joint was flexed 5 degrees to bring the trunk forward over the lower extremities. The knee and ankle joints remained in their starting positions. The shoulder joint was extended 45 degrees, medially rotated 59 degrees, and abducted 39 degrees (Figure 15-3). The elbow joint was flexed an additional 10 degrees; the forearm supinated 84 degrees; the wrist joint flexed an additional 5 degrees and radially deviated 15 degrees. These motions of the shoulder, elbow, and wrist joints brought the hands into a position to grasp the hand rim. The hand assumed a cylindrical power grip on the hand rim (see Figure 15-2). In doing so, the thumb CMC joint abducted 7 degrees; the MCP joint flexed 33 degrees; and the IP joint flexed 54 degrees. Digits two through five flexed at the MCP, PIP, and DIP joints. From second to fifth digit, the MCP joints flexed 69, 72, 83, and 88 degrees, respectively. The PIP joints flexed 57, 65, 73, and 76 degrees, respectively. The DIP joints flexed 48, 53, 53, and 55 degrees, respectively. The subject was now in position to begin propelling the wheelchair forward.[1,15]

As the trunk was brought forward, the erector spinae muscles and the gluteus maximus muscle worked eccentrically to control the forward progression of the trunk. The rectus capitis posterior, oblique capitus, splenius capitis and cervicis, semispinalis capitis and cervicis, and iliocostalis cervicis muscles worked concentrically to extend the neck.[1]

Figure 15-3. Posterior view of reaching for the hand rims: The shoulder joint abducted as the subject reached for the posterior aspect of the hand rim. The key landmarks denoted by black dots are: H = ulnar styloid process (ulnar aspect); I = fifth MCP joint line (ulnar aspect); J = olecranon process; and K = medial epicondyle of humerus.

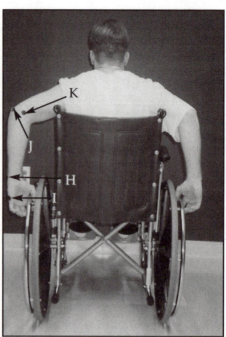

The shoulder joint motion was brought about through concentric activity of the trapezius, rhomboids major and minor, latissimus dorsi, posterior deltoid, teres major, subscapularis, pectoralis major, middle deltoid, and supraspinatus muscles. These muscles worked to extend, medially rotate, and abduct the shoulder joint.[1,28]

The biceps brachii and the triceps brachii muscles worked synergistically to control the motion of the elbow joint. The supinator muscle worked along with the biceps brachii muscle to control the supination of the forearm. The wrist flexion was brought about by concentric activity of the flexors carpi radialis and ulnaris, with the radialis component contributing more due to the radial deviation that occurred.[1,29]

The flexor digitorum profundus, interossei, adductor pollicis, opponens pollicis, and opponens digiti minimi muscles worked concentrically to secure the cylindrical grip around the hand rim.[1,30-31]

PROPELLING THE WHEELCHAIR FORWARD

As the subject began to propel the wheelchair forward (Figure 15-4), the neck remained in the same position of 15 degrees of extension to keep the line of progression in sight. The trunk was brought forward as a whole as the hip flexed an additional 30 degrees. The knee and ankle joints remained in their original positions. The shoulder joint flexed 51 degrees, adducted 54 degrees, and laterally rotated 10 degrees. Initially, the elbow joint flexed an additional 17 degrees. As the forward motion was continued, the elbow joint extended 40 degrees. The forearm pronated 10 degrees. The wrist joint extended 10 degrees and ulnarly deviated back to neutral. The digits of the hand maintained their cylindrical grip on the hand rim, with no change in range of motion.[1,6-7,32-36]

The elbow joint underwent both flexion and extension because the hand was initially positioned below the subject's hip joint. As the subject pushed the wheel forward, the hand came to lie above and then below the hip joint. Since the subject's hand maintained its grip the entire time, this upward and downward motion of the hand was brought about by the flexion and extension motions of the elbow joint.[1,6-7,33]

The ulnar deviation of the wrist optimized the force of the long finger flexors because the heavier an object is, the more likely it is that the wrist will ulnarly deviate.[1,6-7,33,36]

As the subject began to propel the wheelchair forward, the erector spinae muscles worked isometrically to maintain the vertical alignment of the vertebral column. The gluteus maximus muscles worked eccentrically to flex the hip joints, bringing the trunk forward over the lower extremities as the upper extremities were brought forward. The neck extensors worked isometrically to maintain cervical extension.[1,15,37]

The trapezius, levator scapulae, serratus anterior, anterior and middle deltoid, supraspinatus, infraspinatus, teres minor, and pectoralis major muscles worked concentrically to flex, laterally rotate, and adduct the shoulder joint. The biceps brachii, brachialis, and brachioradialis muscles worked concentrically during the first half of the propulsion movement to flex the elbow. The triceps brachii muscle then worked concentrically to complete the extension of the elbow as the wheel was forced forward and downward. The pronators teres and quadratus acted concentrically to pronate the forearm. The extensor carpi ulnaris muscle worked concentrically to extend and ulnarly deviate the wrist joint. The flexors digitorum superficialis and profundus, interossei, adductor pollicis, flexors pollicis longus and brevis, opponens pollicis, and opponens digiti minimi muscles worked isometrically to maintain the grip on the hand rim as the wheel was propelled forward under the weight of the subject's body.[1,15]

Figure 15-4. Propelling the wheelchair forward: The subject pushed the wheels forward using upper extremity and trunk musculature. The key landmarks denoted by black dots are: A = acromion process; B = greater tuberosity of humerus; C = lateral epicondyle of humerus; D = ulnar head (dorsal aspect); H = ulnar styloid process (ulnar aspect); I = fifth MCP joint line (ulnar aspect); J = olecranon process; M = lateral epicondyle of femur; N = fibular head; P = lateral malleolus; R = fifth MTT joint line (lateral aspect); V = greater trochanter of femur; and W = spinous process of C-7.

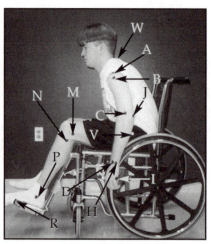

As this phase was completed, there was a loosening of the cylindrical power grip as the upper extremity was brought backward to reposition it for the next forward propulsion of the wheelchair. During this time, the digits were extended and abducted as they prepared to regrip the hand rim. The extension and abduction ranges of motion were proportional to the flexion and adduction ranges at the beginning of this activity.

The extensors digitorum, indicis, digiti minimi, and pollicis longus and brevis, abductors pollicis longus and brevis, and the interossei muscles worked concentrically to reposition the hand to resume the grip on the hand rim. Once the hand was repositioned, the activity described previously alternated back and forth to continue forward propulsion of the wheelchair.[1,15,21,31]

CONTINUING THE PROPULSION FORWARD

For the remaining forward propulsion, the subject alternated back and forth between bringing the upper extremities in back of the trunk (to regrasp the hand rims and prepare for the next forward propulsion of the wheelchair) and moving the upper extremities in front of the trunk (to propel the wheelchair forward).[1]

SUMMARY

Key Anatomical Landmarks for Wheelchair Analysis

Shoulder Complex:	Acromion process
	Greater tuberosity of humerus
Elbow and Forearm Complex:	Lateral epicondyle of humerus
	Medial epicondyle of humerus
	Olecranon process
	Radial styloid process (dorsal aspect)
	Radial styloid process (radial aspect)
	Ulnar head (dorsal aspect)
	Ulnar styloid process (ulnar aspect)
Wrist and Hand Complex:	Base of first MCP (radial and dorsal aspects)
	Base of second MCP (radial aspect)
	Base of fifth MCP (ulnar aspect)
	First MCP joint line (dorsal and radial aspects)
	Second MCP joint line (radial aspect)
	Fifth MCP joint line (ulnar aspect)
	First IP joint line (radial aspect)
	Second PIP joint line (radial aspect)
	Fifth PIP joint line (ulnar aspect)
	Second DIP joint line (radial aspect)
	Fifth DIP joint line (ulnar aspect)
Hip Complex:	Greater trochanter of femur
Knee Complex:	Lateral epicondyle of femur
	Fibular head
Ankle and Foot Complex:	Lateral malleolus
	Fifth MTT joint line (lateral aspect)
Spinal Complex:	Spinous process of C-7
	Spinous process of T-12
	Spinous process of L-5

Major Phases for Wheelchair Analysis

Starting Position

- Position of subject

- Description of wheelchair

Reaching for the Hand Rims

Propelling the Wheelchair Forward

Continuing the Propulsion Forward

Joint Motions and Muscular Activity: Propelling a Wheelchair

Introduction and Set-Up

- Cervical region in forward flexion, with thoracolumbar region in neutral.

- Shoulder joint in internal rotation, with elbow and wrist joints flexed.

- Radioulnar joints pronated.

- Digits primarily in flexion.

- Hip and knee joints flexed, with ankles in neutral.

Reaching for the Hand Rims

- Cervical region and shoulder joints in extension.

- Elbow and wrist joints in flexion and radioulnar joints in supination.

- Digits in flexion primarily.

- Hip joints in flexion.

- Concentric muscular contractions for all motions.

- All other joints are maintaining their positions.

Propelling the Wheelchair Forward

- Shoulder and elbow joints in flexion.

- Radioulnar joints in pronation.

- Wrist joints in extension and ulnar deviation.

- Hips in flexion.

- Concentric muscular contractions for all motions.

- All other joints are maintaining their positions.

Continuing the Propulsion Forward

- Motions alternate back and forth between bringing both upper extremities in back of the trunk and moving both upper extremities in front of the trunk (regrasping the hand rims and propelling forward).

CLINICAL APPLICATION AND DISCUSSION QUESTIONS

The analysis in this chapter focused on a standard wheelchair being propelled forward. Repeat this analysis from the perspective of propelling the wheelchair backward. Compare the motions and the muscular activity, then do the analysis from the perspective of turning the wheelchair in a circle.

In the analysis presented in this chapter, the subject was capable of maintaining erect posture when seated. Compare this analysis to the individual who has difficulty maintaining normal erect posture.

Next, compare this analysis to one using a racing wheelchair. Think about body posture given the design of a racing chair. What changes will be seen in the upper extremity muscular activity?

How will the analysis change for a bilateral lower extremity amputee? What wheelchair modifications will be needed to account for the weight loss of the lower extremities?

What wheelchair modifications could be made for an individual with hand grasp problems? How would these modifications affect the muscular activity of the upper extremities when propelling the wheelchair? What modifications would be needed for an individual who can use only one upper extremity to control the wheelchair?

Do an analysis of maneuvering a wheelchair through a doorway, including opening the door. How did the analysis change from that of propelling the wheelchair in a straight line without having to negotiate a doorway or open a door?

Finally, make a list of muscle substitutions that could be used for the muscles cited in this analysis. Compare it to Charts 1 through 3 in Appendix A.

REFERENCES

1. Lamontagne M. Biomechanical study of wheelchair propulsion. In: G de Groot, AH Hollander, PA Hujing, GJ van Ingen Schenau, eds. *Biomechanics X1-A: International Series on Biomechanics, 7-A*. Amsterdam, Holland: Free University Press; 1987.

2. Andersson GBJ, Ortengren R. Lumbar disc pressure and myoelectric back muscle activity during sitting. III. Studies on a wheelchair. *Scand J Rehabil Med*. 1974;6:122-127.

3. Lucas DB, Bresler B. *Stability of the Ligamentous Spine*. Report *Number 40*. San Francisco, Calif: University of California Biomechanics Laboratory.

4. Lucas DB. Mechanics of the spine. *Bull Hosp Jt Dis*. 1970;31:115-131.

5. Howorth B. The painful coccyx. *Journal of the West Pacific Orthopedic Association*. 1978;15:39-56.

6. Jones FP, Gray FE, Hanson JA, Shoop JD. Neck muscle tension and the postural image. *Ergonomics*. 1961;4:133-142.

7. Gray FE, Hanson JA, Jones FP. Postural aspects of neck muscle tension. *Ergonomics*. 1966;9:245-256.

8. Hughes CJ, Weimar WH, Sheth PN. Biomechanics of wheelchair propulsion as a function of seat position and user-to-chair interface. *Arch Phys Med Rehabil*. 1992;73:263-269.

9. Brattgard SO. Design of wheelchairs and wheelchair service based on scientific research. *Readaptation*. 1969;11:162-172.

10. Brunswic M. Ergonomics of seat design. *Physiother*. 1984;70:40-43.

11. Engel P, Hildebrandt G. Wheelchair design—technological and physiological aspects. *Proceedings of the Royal Society of Medicine*. 1974;67:409-413.

12. Loane TH, Kirby RL. Static rear stability of conventional and lightweight variable-axle-position wheelchairs. *Arch Phys Med Rehabil*. 1985;66:174-176.

13. Andersson GBJ, Murphy RW, Ortengren R, Nachemson AL. The influence of backrest inclination and lumbar support on the lumbar lordosis in sitting. *Spine*. 1979;4:52-58.

14. Platts EA. Wheelchair design—survey of users' views. *Proceedings of the Royal Society of Medicine*. 1974;67:414-416.

15. van der Woude LHV, de Groot G, Hollander AP, van Ingen Schenau GJ, Rozendal RH. Wheelchair ergonomics and physiological testing of prototypes. *Ergonomics.* 1986;29:1561-1573.

16. Gracovetsky S, Farfan H. The optimum spine. *Spine.* 1986;11:543-573.

17. Ålund M, Larsson SE. Three-dimensional analysis of neck motion: a clinical method. *Spine.* 1990;15:87-91.

18. Blakely RL, Palmer ML. Analysis of rotation accompanying shoulder flexion. *Phys Ther.* 1984;64:1214-1216.

19. London JT. Kinematics of the elbow. *J Bone Joint Surg Am.* 1981;63:529-535.

20. Wadsworth CT. Clinical anatomy and mechanics of the wrist and hand. *J Orthop Sports Phys Ther.* 1983;4:206-216.

21. An KN, Chao EY, Cooney WP, Linscheid RI. Normative model of human hand for biomechanical analysis. *J Biomech.* 1979;12:775-788.

22. Radin EL. Biomechanics of the human hip. *Clin Orthop.* 1980;152:28-34.

23. Blackburn TA, Craig E. Knee anatomy: a brief review. *Phys Ther.* 1980;60:1556-1560.

24. Donatelli R. Normal biomechanics of the foot and ankle. *J Orthop Sports Phys Ther.* 1985;7:91-95.

25. Andersson GBJ, Johnson B, Ortengren R. Myoelectric activity in individual lumbar erector spinae muscles during sitting: a study with surface and wire electrodes. *Scand J Rehabil Med.* 1974;3(suppl):91-108.

26. Andersson GBJ, Ortengren R. Myoelectric back muscle activity during sitting. *Scand J Rehab Med.* 1974;3(suppl):73-90.

27. Andersson GBJ, Ortengren R, Nachemson AL. The sitting posture: an electromyographic and discometric study. *Orthop Clin North Am.* 1975;6:105-120.

28. Kronberg M, Nemeth G, Brostrom L. Muscle activity and coordination in the normal shoulder. *Clin Orthop.* 1990;257:76-85.

29. Boninger ML, Cooper RA, Robertson RN. Wrist biomechanics during two speeds of wheelchair propulsion: an analysis using a local coordinate system. *Arch Phys Med Rehabil.* 1997;78:364-372.

30. Jones LA. The assessment of hand function: a critical review of techniques. *J Hand Surg Am.* 1989;14:221-228.

31. Landsmeer JMF. Power grip and precision handling. *Ann Rheum Dis.* 1962;21:164-170.

32. Chari VR, Kirby RL. Lower-limb influence on sitting balance while reaching forward. *Arch Phys Med Rehabil.* 1986;67:730-733.

33. Wang YT, Deutsch H, Morse M. Three-dimensional kinematics of wheelchair propulsion across racing speeds. *Adapted Physical Activity Quarterly.* 1995;12:78-89.

34. Davis JL, Browney ES, Jonson ME, Iuliano BA, An K. Three-dimensional kinematics of the shoulder complex during wheelchair propulsion: a technical report. *J Rehabil Res Dev.* 1998;35:61-72.

35. Veeger HEJ, van der Helm FCT, Rozendal RH. Orientation of the scapula in a simulated wheelchair push. *Clin Biomech*. 1993;8:81-90.

36. Youm Y, McMurty RY, Flatt AE, Gillespie TE. Kinematics of the wrist. I. An experimental study of radial-ulnar deviation and flexion-extension. *J Bone Joint Surg Am*. 1978;60:423-432.

37. Joseph J, McColl I. Electromyography of muscles of posture: posterior vertebral muscles in males. *J Physiol (Lond)*. 1961;157:33-37.

SUGGESTED READINGS

Andersson GBJ, Ortengren R, Nachemson A, Elfstrom G. Lumbar disc pressure and myoelectric back muscle activity during sitting. I. Studies on an experimental chair. *Scand J Rehabil Med*. 1974;6:104-114.

Atkeson CG. Learning arm kinematics and dynamics. *Annu Rev Neurosci*. 1989;12:157-183.

Ayoub MM, LoPresti P. The determination of an optimum size cylindrical handle by use of electromyography. *Ergonomics*. 1971;4:503-518.

Burnham RS. Shoulder pain in wheelchair athletes. *Am J Sports Med*. 1993;21:238-242.

Engen TJ, Spencer WA. Method of kinematic study of normal upper extremity movements. *Arch Phys Med Rehabil*. 1968;49:9-11.

Herberts P, Kadefors R, Broman H. Arm positioning in manual tasks—an electromyographic study of localized muscle fatigue. *Ergonomics*. 1980;23:655-665.

Jonsson B. The functions of individual muscles in the lumbar part of the spinal muscle. *Electromyography*. 1970;10:5-21.

Mayall JK, Desharnais G. *Positioning in a Wheelchair*. Thorofare, NJ: SLACK Incorporated; 1990.

Nolan JP, Sherk HH. Biomechanical evaluation of the extensor musculature of the cervical spine. *Spine*. 1988;13:9-11.

Panjabi M, Abumi K, Duranceau J, Oxland T. Spinal stability and intersegmetal muscle forces: a biomechanical model. *Spine*. 1989;14:194-200.

Pope PM. A study of instability in relation to posture in the wheelchair. *Physiother*. 1985;72:124-129.

Radonjic D, Long CL. Kinesiology of the wrist. *Am J Phys Med Rehabil*. 1971;50:57-71.

Rodgers MM, Gayle GW, Figoni SF. Biomechanics of wheelchair propulsion during fatigue. *Arch Phys Med Rehabil*. 1994;75:85-93.

Rydell N. Biomechanics of the hip joint. *Clin Orthop*. 1973;92:6-15.

Stroyan M, Wilk KE. The functional anatomy of the elbow complex. *J Orthop Sports Phys Ther*. 1993;17:279-288.

Warren CG, Ko M, Smith C, Imre JV. Reducing back displacement in the powered reclining wheelchair. *Arch Phys Med Rehabil.* 1982;63:447-449.

White AA, Johnson RM, Panjabi MM, Southwick WO. Biomechanical analysis of clinical stability in the cervical spine. *Clin Orthop.* 1975;109:85-96.

Charts of Prime Muscles for Body Motion and Possible Substitutions

Chart 1
Upper Extremity Muscles—Prime Movers and Possible Substitutions

Joint	Motion	Normal Muscles	Substitute Muscles*
Scapulo-thoracic	Elevation	Upper trapezius Levator scapulae	Rhomboids major and minor
	Adduction	Middle trapezius Rhomboids major and minor	Posterior deltoid Latissimus dorsi
	Adduction and depression	Lower trapezius	Latissimus dorsi Pectoralis major and minor Latissimus dorsi Levator scapulae
	Abduction and upward rotation	Serratus anterior	Upper trapezius
Shoulder	Flexion	Anterior deltoid Coracobrachialis	Biceps brachii—long head Upper trapezius Pectoralis major
	Extension	Latissimus dorsi Teres major Posterior deltoid	Triceps brachii—long head
	Abduction	Middle deltoid Supraspinatus	Biceps brachii—long head
	Horizontal abduction	Posterior deltoid	Triceps brachii—long head
	Horizontal adduction	Pectoralis major Anterior deltoid	Coracobrachialis
	Medial rotation	Subscapularis Pectoralis major Latissimus dorsi Teres major	Anterior deltoid
	Lateral rotation	Infraspinatus Teres minor	Posterior deltoid

* Note: When muscles are substituted for the prime movers, the pure joint motion will not occur or the joint motion will be weak.

Chart 1 (continued)

Upper Extremity Muscles—Prime Movers and Possible Substitutions

Joint	Motion	Normal Muscles	Substitute Muscles
Elbow	Flexion	Biceps brachii Brachialis Brachioradialis	Flexor carpi ulnaris Flexor carpi radialis
	Extension	Triceps brachii Anconeus	Extensor carpi ulnaris Extensors carpi radialii longus and brevis
Forearm	Pronation	Pronator teres Pronator quadratus	Brachioradialis
	Supination	Biceps brachii Supinator	Brachioradialis
Wrist	Flexion	Flexor carpi radialis Flexor carpi ulnaris	Flexor digitorum superficialis Flexor digitorum profundus Palmaris longus Abductor pollicis longus Flexor pollicis longus
	Extension	Extensor carpi ulnaris Extensor carpi radialii longus and brevis	Extensor digitorum Extensor indicis Extensor digiti minimi Extensor pollicis longus
	Ulnar deviation	Flexor carpi ulnaris Extensor carpi ulnaris	
	Radial deviation	Flexor carpi radialis Extensors carpi radialii longus and brevis	
Thumb	Carpometa-carpal opposition	Opponens pollicis	Adductor pollicis Flexors pollicis longus and brevis Abductor pollicis brevis
	Metacarpo-phalangeal flexion	Flexor pollicis brevis	Flexor pollicis longus
	Metacarpo-phalangeal extension	Extensor pollicis brevis	Extensor pollicis longus

Chart 1 (continued)
Upper Extremity Muscles—Prime Movers and Possible Substitutions

Joint	Motion	Normal Muscles	Substitute Muscles
	Inter-phalangeal extension	Extensor pollicis longus	Abductor pollicis brevis Flexor pollicis brevis Adductor pollicis (working together)
	Abduction	Abductors pollicis longus and brevis	Extensors pollicis longus and brevis Palmaris longus
	Adduction	Adductor pollicis	Flexors pollicis longus and brevis Extensor pollicis longus First dorsal interosseous
Digits 2 through 5	Metacarpo-phalangeal flexion	Lumbricals Dorsal interossei Palmar interossei	Flexor digitorum superficialis and profundus
	Proximal inter-phalangeal flexion	Flexor digitorum superficialis	Flexor digitorum profundus
	Distal inter-phalangeal flexion	Flexor digitorum profundus	
	Extension	Extensors digitorum, indicis, and digiti minimi	
	Abduction	Dorsal interossei Abductor digiti minimi	
	Adduction	Palmar interossei	
Digit 5	Opposition	Opponens digiti minimi	

Chart 2
Lower Extremity Muscles—Prime Movers and Possible Substitutions

Joint	Motion	Normal Muscles	Substitute Muscles*
Hip	Flexion	Iliopsoas	Sartorius Rectus femoris Hip lateral rotators Pectineus
	Flexion, abduction, and lateral rotation	Sartorius	Iliopsoas Rectus femoris
	Extension	Gluteus maximus Semitendinosus Semimembranosus Biceps femoris—long head	
	Abduction	Glutei medius and minimus	Tensor fasciae latae Hip flexors Quadratus lumborum Gluteus maximus—upper fibers
	Abduction with flexion	Tensor fasciae latae	Hip flexors Glutei medius and minimus
	Adduction	Adductors magnus, longus and brevis Pectineus Gracilis	Hip flexors Hamstrings
	Medial rotation	Tensor fasciae latae Gluteus minimus Gluteus medius	
	Lateral rotation	Piriformis Gemelii superior and inferior Obturators internus and externus Quadratus femoris	Gluteus maximus—posterior fibers

* Note: When muscles are substituted for the prime movers, the pure joint motion will not occur or the joint motion will be weak.

Chart 2 (continued)

Lower Extremity Muscles—Prime Movers and Possible Substitutions

Joint	Motion	Normal Muscles	Substitute Muscles
Knee	Flexion	Biceps femoris Semitendinous Semimembranosus	Hip flexors Sartorius Gracilis Gastrocnemius
	Extension	Quadriceps femoris	Hip internal rotators (in sidelying position only)
Ankle	Dorsiflexion	Tibialis anterior	Extensor hallicus longus Extensor digitorum longus
	Plantarflexion	Gastrocnemius soleus	Posterior tibialis Flexor hallucis longus Flexor digitorum longus Peronei longus and brevis
Subtalar	Inversion	Tibialis posterior	Flexor digitorum longus Flexor hallucis longus Tibialis anterior
	·Eversion	Peronei longus, brevis, and tertius	Peroneus tertius Extensor digitorum longus
Digits 1 through 5	Metatarso- phalangeal flexion	Lumbricals Flexor hallucis brevis	Flexors digitorum longus and brevis Flexor hallucis longus Flexor digiti minimi
	Metatarso- phalangeal extension	Extensors digitorum longus and brevis	
	Inter- phalangeal flexion	Flexors digitorum longus and brevis Flexor hallucis longus	
	Inter- phalangeal extension	Extensors digitorum longus and brevis Extensor hallucis longus	

Chart 3
Neck and Trunk Muscles—Prime Movers and Possible Substitutions

Joint	Motion	Normal Muscles	Substitute Muscles*
Neck	Flexion	Longus capitis Longus colli Rectus capitis anterior and lateralis Scalenus anterior, medial, and posterior Sternocleidomastoid	Sternocleidomastoid
	Anterolateral flexion	Sternocleidomastoid	
	Extension	Rectus capitis Posterior major and minor Longissimus capitis and cervicis Oblique capitis superior and inferior Splenius capitis and cervicis	Upper trapezius
Trunk	Flexion	Rectus abdominis	Internal abdominal oblique External abdominal oblique Psoas major and minor
	Extension	Erector spinae— thoracic and lumbar components Multifidus Semispinalis thoracis Quadratus lumborum	
	Rotation	External and internal abdominal obliques	Latissimus dorsi Rectus abdominis Deep back muscles (one side)

* Note: When muscles are substituted for the prime movers, the pure joint motion will not occur or the joint motion will be weak.

Chart 3 (continued)
Neck and Trunk Muscles—Prime Movers and Possible Substitutions

Joint	Motion	Normal Muscles	Substitute Muscles*
Pelvis	Elevation	Quadratus lumborum	Latissimus dorsi Oblique external abdominal Oblique internal abdominal Iliocostalis lumborum

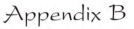

Appendix B

Suggested Textbook Readings

Akkas N, ed. *Progress in Biomechanics.* Alphen aan den Rijn, Netherlands: Sijthoff and Noordhoof; 1979.

Alexander RM. *Animal Mechanics.* Seattle, Wash: University of Washington Press; 1986.

Alexander MR. *The Human Machine.* Irvington, NY: Columbia University Press; 1992.

American Academy of Orthopaedic Surgeons. *Joint Motion—Method of Measuring and Recording.* Chicago, Ill: American Academy of Orthopaedic Surgeons; 1965.

Anderson T. *Human Kinetics and Analyzing Body Movements.* London, England: William Heinemann Ltd; 1951.

Baines RM. *Motion and Time Study: Design and Measurement of Work.* 7th ed. Somerset, NJ: John Wiley & Sons Inc; 1980.

Barnham JN. *Mechanical Kinesiology.* St. Louis, Mo: CV Mosby; 1978.

Basmajian JV, DeLuca C. *Muscles Alive, Their Functions Revealed by Electromyography.* Baltimore, Md: Williams & Wilkins Co; 1985.

Berme N, Cappozzo A, eds. *Biomechanics of Human Movement: Applications in Rehabilitation, Sports, and Ergonomics.* Worthington, Ohio: Bertec Corp; 1990.

Berryman N. *Muscle and Sensory Testing.* Philadelphia, Pa: WB Saunders Co; 1999.

Black S. *Man and Motor Cars.* New York, NY: WW Norton & Co Inc; 1966.

Broer MR, Zernicke RF. *Efficiency of Human Movement.* Philadelphia, Pa: WB Saunders Co; 1979.

Brown LS, ed. *Animals in Motion.* Mineola, NY: Dover Publications; 1957.

Brubaker CE, McClay IS, McLaurin CA. Effect of seat position on wheelchair propulsion efficiency. In: *Proceedings of the Second International Conference on Rehabilitation Engineering.* Ottawa, Canada: 1984:12-14.

Bruer J. *A Handbook of Assistive Devices for the Handicapped Elderly—New Help for Individual Living.* Binghamton, NY: Haworth Press Inc; 1982.

Brunnstrom S. *Clinical Kinesiology*. 3rd ed. Philadelphia, Pa: FA Davis Co; 1972.

Bulstrode S, Harrison RA, Clarke AK. *Assessment of Back Rests for Use in Car Seats*. Lancashire, UK: DHSS Aids Assessment Programme, Health Publications Unit; 1983.

Burke RK, Rasch P. *Kinesiology of Applied Anatomy*. Philadelphia, Pa: Lea & Febiger; 1975.

Burstein AH, Wright TM. *Fundamentals of Orthopaedic Biomechanics*. Baltimore, Md: Williams & Wilkins Co; 1994.

Carlsöö S. *How Man Moves*. London, England: William Heinemann Ltd; 1972.

Cavanaugh RP, Irvin FE. *The Physiology and Biomechanics of Cycling*. Somerset, NJ: John Wiley & Sons Inc; 1978.

Chaffin DB, Andersson GBJ. *Occupational Biomechanics*. 2nd ed. Somerset, NJ: John Wiley & Sons Inc; 1991.

Chaffin DB. Biomechanics of manual materials handling and low-back pain. In C Zenz, ed. *Occupational Medicine*. Chicago, Ill: Year Book; 1975:443-467.

Cheng IS. *Computer-Television Analysis of Biped Locomotion*. Columbus, Ohio: Ohio State University; 1974. Thesis.

Claiborne DK. *Ergonomics and Cumulative Trauma Disorders: A Handbook for Occupational Therapists*. San Diego, Calif: Singular Publishing Group; 1999.

Close JD. *Functional Anatomy of the Extremities*. Springfield, Ill: Charles C. Thomas Publishing; 1973.

Cochran GVB. *A Primer of Orthopedic Biomechanics*. New York, NY: Churchill Livingstone; 1982.

Cooper JM, Glassow RB. *Kinesiology*. 2nd ed. St. Louis, Mo: The CV Mosby Co; 1976.

Cooper RA. *Wheelchair Selection and Configuration*. New York, NY: Demos; 1998.

Damodaran L, Simpson A, Wilson P. *Designing Systems for People*. Manchester, England: NCC Publications; 1980.

Damon A, Stoudt HW, McFarland RA. *The Human Body in Equipment Design*. Cambridge, Mass: Harvard University Press; 1966.

Dempster WT. Free body diagrams as an approach to the mechanics of posture and motion. In: FG Evans, ed. *Biomechanical Studies of the Musculoskeletal System*. Springfield, Ill: Charles C. Thomas Publisher; 1961.

Enoka RM. *Neuromechanical Basis of Kinesiology*. 2nd ed. Champaign, Ill: Human Kinetics Publishers Inc; 1994.

Esch D, Lepley M. *Evaluation of Joint Motion: Methods of Measurement and Recording*. Minneapolis, Minn: University of Minnesota Press; 1974.

Eshkol N, Wachman A. *Movement Notation*. London, England: Weidefeld & Nicholson; 1958.

Fenwick D. *Wheelchairs and Their Users*. London, England: HMSO; 1977.

Frankel VH, Burstein AH. *Orthopedic Biomechanics*. Philadelphia, Pa: Lea & Febiger; 1970.

Frankel VH, Nordin M. *Basic Biomechanics of the Skeletal System.* Philadelphia, Pa: Lea & Febiger; 1980.

Frost HM. *An Introduction to Biomechanics.* Springfield, Ill: Charles C. Thomas; 1967.

Galley PM, Forster AL. *Human Movement: An Introductory Text for Physiotherapy Students.* 2nd ed. New York, NY: Churchill Livingstone; 1987.

Goldberg B, Hsu JD, eds. *Atlas of Orthoses and Assistive Devices.* 3rd ed. St. Louis, Mo: Mosby; 1997.

Goldthwait JE, Brown LT, Swaim LT, Kuhns JG. *Essentials of Body Mechanics in Health and Disease.* 5th ed. Philadelphia, Pa: JB Lippincott Co; 1952.

Gowitzke BA, Milner M. *Scientific Basis of Human Movement.* 3rd ed. Baltimore, Md: Williams & Wilkins Company; 1988.

Grandjean E. *Ergonomics of the Home.* London, England: Taylor & Francis; 1973.

Grandjean E. Sitting posture of car drivers from the point of view of ergonomics. In: DJ Oborne, JA Levis, eds. *Human Factors in Transport Research.* Vol. 2. London, England: Academic Press; 1980b:205-213.

Grieve DW, Miller DI, Mitchelson D, Paul JP, Smith AJ. *Techniques for the Analysis of Human Movement.* Princeton, NJ: Princeton Book Co; 1976.

Hall SJ. *Basic Biomechanics.* 2nd ed. St. Louis, Mo: Mosby; 1995.

Hamill J, Knutzen KM. *Biomechanical Basis of Human Movement.* Baltimore, Md: Williams & Wilkins Co; 1995.

Hay JG, Reid JG. *The Anatomical and Mechanical Basis of Human Motion.* Englewood Cliffs, NJ: Prentice Hall Inc; 1988.

Hollinshead WH. *Functional Anatomy of the Limbs and Back.* 4th ed. Philadelphia, Pa: WB Saunders Co; 1976.

Inman VT. *Joints of the Ankle.* Baltimore, Md: Williams & Wilkins Co; 1976.

Jensen CR, Schultz GW. *Applied Kinesiology.* New York, NY: McGraw-Hill Inc; 1970.

Joseph J. *Man's Posture, Electromyographic Studies.* Springfield, Ill: Charles C. Thomas Publisher; 1960.

Junghanns H. *Clinical Implications of Normal Biomechanical Stresses on Spinal Function.* Rockville, Md: Aspen Publishers Inc; 1990.

Jürgens HW. Body movements of the driver in relation to sitting conditions in the car: a methodological study. In: DJ Oborne, JA Levis, eds. *Human Factors in Transport Research.* Vol. 2. London, England: Academic Press; 1980:249-256.

Kane TR, Levinson DA. *Dynamics: Theory and Application.* New York, NY: McGraw-Hill Inc; 1985.

Kelsey JL, Harris P, Koreiger N. *Upper Extremity Disorders: A Survey of Their Frequency and Cost in the United States.* St. Louis, Mo: CV Mosby Co; 1980.

Kendall FP, McCreary EK, Provance PG. *Muscles—Testing and Function.* 4th ed. Baltimore, Md: Williams & Wilkins; 1993.

Klein-Vogelbach S. *Functional Kinetics—Observing, Analyzing, and Teaching Human Movement*. Berlin, Germany: Springer-Verlag; 1990.

Koff DG. Joint kinematics. Camera-based approach. In: RL Craik, CA Oatis, eds. *Gait Analysis*. St. Louis, Mo: Mosby; 1995: 183-204.

Kreighbaum E, Barthels K. *Biomechanics: A Qualitative Approach for Studying Human Movement*. Tappan, NJ: Allyn & Bacon; 1996.

Lehmkuhl LD, Smith LK. *Brunnstrom's Clinical Kinesiology*. 4th ed. Philadelphia, Pa: FA Davis Co; 1984.

LeVeau B, ed. *Biomechanics of Human Motion*. Philadelphia, Pa: WB Saunders; 1977.

Luttgrens K, Deutsch H, Hamilton N. *Kinesiology: Scientific Basis of Human Motion*. 8th ed. Dubuque, Iowa: Brown & Benchmark; 1992.

MacConaill MA, Basmajian JV. *Muscles and Movements: A Basis for Human Kinesiology*. Baltimore, Md: Williams & Wilkins Co; 1969.

Mayall JK, Desharnais G. *Positioning in a Wheelchair*. Thorofare, NJ: SLACK Incorporated; 1990.

Maybridge E. *The Male and Female Figure in Motion*. Mineola, NY: Dover Publications; 1984.

Merian JL. *Dynamics*. Somerset, NJ: John Wiley & Sons Inc; 1975.

Miller DI, Nelson RC. *Biomechanics of Sport*. Philadelphia, Pa: Lea & Febiger; 1973.

Mital A, Karwowski W, eds. *Ergonomics in Rehabilitation*. Philadelphia, Pa: Taylor & Francis Inc; 1988.

Moore KL. *Clinically Oriented Anatomy*. 3rd ed. Baltimore, Md: Williams & Wilkins Co; 1992.

Morecki A, ed. *Biomechanics of Engineering: Modeling, Simulation, Control*. New York, NY: Springer-Verlag; 1987.

Muybridge E. *The Human Figure in Motion*. Mineola, NY: Dover Publications; 1955.

Nahum AM, Melvin JW, eds. *Accidental Injury: Biomechanics and Prevention*. New York, NY: Springer-Verlag; 1993.

NIOSH. *Work Practices Guide for Manual Lifting*. Cincinnati, Ohio: DHHS Publication No.81-122; 1981.

Norkin CC, Levangie PK. *Joint Structure and Function: A Comprehensive Analysis*. 2nd ed. Philadelphia, Pa: FA Davis Co; 1992.

Norkin J, Frankel V. *Basic Biomechanics of the Musculoskeletal System*. Philadelphia, Pa: Lea & Febiger; 1989.

Oliver J, Middleditch A. *Functional Anatomy of the Spine*. Oxford, England: Butterworth-Heinemann Ltd; 1991.

Palastanga N, Field D, Soames R. *Anatomy and Human Movement—Structure and Function*. 2nd ed. Oxford, England: Butterworth-Heinemann Ltd; 1994.

Palmer ML, Epler M. *Clinical Assessment Procedures in Physical Therapy*. Philadelphia, Pa: JB Lippincott Co; 1990.

Pauwels F. *Biomechanics of the Normal and Disease Hip*. Berlin, Germany: Springer-Verlag; 1976.

Peterson N, Bownas D. Skill, task structure, and performance acquisition. In: M Dunnette, EA Fleishman, eds. *Human Performance and Productivity, Vol. 1— Human Capability Assessment*. Hillsdale, NJ: Earlbaum Associates; 1982:49-105.

Plagenhoef S. *Patterns of Human Motion: A Cinematographic Analysis*. Englewood Cliffs, NJ: Prentice Hall; 1971.

Pletta DH, Frederick D. *Engineering Mechanics, Statics, and Dynamics*. New York, NY: The Ronald Press; 1964.

Powell ME. *Trunk Strength and Flexibility as Factors in Posture*. Wellesley, Mass: Wellesley College; 1930. Thesis.

Radin EL, Rose RM, Blaha DJ, Litsky AS. *Practical Biomechanics for the Orthopedic Surgeon*. 2nd ed. New York, NY: Churchill Livingstone Inc; 1992.

Rasch PJ, Burke RK. *Kinesiology and Applied Anatomy*. Philadelphia, Pa: Lea & Febiger; 1978.

Reese NB. *Muscle and Sensory Testing*. Philadelphia, Pa: WB Saunders Co; 1999.

Reid G, Hay J. *The Anatomical and Mechanical Basis of Human Motion*. Englewoods Cliff, NJ: Prentice Hall Inc; 1982.

Roberts SL, Falkenburg SA. *Biomechanics: Problem Solving for Functional Activity*. St. Louis, Mo: Mosby-Year Book Inc; 1992.

Robertson LR. *Injuries: Causes, Control Strategies, and Public Policy*. Lexington, Mass: Lexington Books; 1983.

Root ML, Orient WP, Weed JH. *Normal and Abnormal Function of the Foot: Clinical Biomechanics, Vol. II*. Los Angeles, Calif: Clinical Biomechanics Corp; 1977.

Rosee C, Clawson DK. *The Musculoskeletal System in Health and Disease*. Hagerstown, Md: Harper & Row; 1980.

Saha AK. *Theory of Shoulder Mechanism: Descriptive and Applied*. Springfield, Ill: Charles C. Thomas Publisher; 1961.

Sanders MS, McCormick EJ. *Human Factors in Engineering and Design*. 7th ed. New York, NY: McGraw-Hill Inc; 1993.

Sarrafian SK. *Anatomy of the Foot and Ankle: Descriptive, Topographic, Functional*. 2nd ed. Philadelphia, Pa: JB Lippincott Co; 1993.

Schafer RC. *Clinical Biomechanics. Musculoskeletal Actions and Reactions*. Baltimore, Md: Williams & Wilkins Co; 1983.

Schenck JM, Cordova FD. *Introductory Biomechanics*. 2nd ed. Philadelphia, Pa: FA Davis Co; 1980.

Scott MG. *Analysis of Human Motion*. New York, NY: Appleton-Century-Crofts; 1963.

Sgarlato TE. *A Compendium of Podiatric Biomechanics*. San Francisco, Calif: College of Podiatric Medicine; 1971.

Singleton WT. *The Body at Work: Biological Ergonomics*. Cambridge, Mass: Cambridge University Press; 1982.

Smith LK, Weiss EL, Lehmkuhl LD, eds. *Brunnstrom's Clinical Kinesiology*. 5th ed. Philadelphia, Pa: FA Davis Co; 1996.

Snell R. *Clinical Anatomy for Medical Students*. 5th ed. Boston, Mass: Little Brown & Co; 1995.

Soderberg GL. *Kinesiology—Application to Pathological Motion*. Baltimore, Md: Williams & Wilkins Co; 1986.

Spinner M. *Kaplan's Functional and Surgical Anatomy of the Hand*. 3rd ed. Philadelphia, Pa: JB Lippincott Co; 1984.

Steindler A. *Kinesiology of the Human Body Under Normal and Pathological Conditions*. Springfield, Ill: Charles C. Thomas Publisher; 1955.

Sweigard LE. *Human Movement Potential: Its Ideokinetic Facilitation*. New York, NY: Harper & Row Inc; 1974.

Tichauer ER. *The Biomechanical Basis of Ergonomics*. Somerset, NJ: John F. Wiley Sons Inc; 1978.

Tyldesley B, Grieve JI. *Muscles, Nerves, and Movement: Kinesiology in Daily Living*. 2nd ed. Oxford, England: Blackwell Science; 1996.

U.S. Department of Health and Human Services.*Promoting Health/Preventing Disease. Year 2000 Objective for the Nation*. Washington, DC: Government Printing Office; 1989.

Watkins J. *An Introduction to Mechanics of Human Movement*. Lancaster, UK: MTP Press Ltd; 1983.

Webb RDG. *Industrial Ergonomics*. Ontario, Canada: The Industrial Accident Prevention Association; 1982.

Wells KF, Luttgrens K. *Kinesiology: Scientific Basis of Human Motion*. Philadelphia, Pa: WB Saunders Co; 1976.

White AA, Panjabi MM. *Clinical Biomechanics of the Spine*. 2nd ed. Philadelphia, Pa: JB Lippincott Co; 1990.

Whiting WC, Zernicke RF. *Biomechanics of Musculoskeletal Injuries*. Champaign, Ill: Human Kinetics Publishers Inc; 1998.

Widule CJ. *Analysis of Human Motion*. West Lafayette, Ind: Balt Publishers; 1974.

Wiktorin CH, Nordin M. *Introduction to Problem Solving in Biomechanics*. Philadelphia, Pa: Lea & Febiger; 1986.

Williams M, Lissner HR. *Biomechanics of Human Motion*. Philadelphia, Pa: WB Saunders Co; 1962.

Winter DA. *Biomechanics and Motor Control of Human Movement*. 2nd ed. New York, NY: John Wiley & Sons Inc; 1990.

Winter DA. *Biomechanics of Human Movement*. New York, NY: John Wiley & Sons Inc; 1979.

Wright V, Ladin ER, eds. *Mechanics of Human Joints*. New York, NY: Marcel Dekker Inc; 1993.

Wright WG. *Muscle Function*. New York, NY: Hafner Publishing Co; 1962.

Zacharow D. *The Healthy Lower Back*. Springfield, Ill: Thomas Publishing; 1984.

Zacharow D. *Posture: Sitting, Standing, Chair Design, and Exercise.* New York, NY: Charles C. Thomas Publishing; 1988.

Zatsjorsky VM. *Kinematics of Human Motion.* Champaign, Ill: Human Kinetics Publishers Inc; 1998.

Zenz C, ed. *Occupational Medicine.* Chicago, Ill: Year Book; 1975.

Index

flexor pollicis muscles
    actions of, 26, 41, 78, 120, 233
        in donning shirt, 63, 69-70
        in driving, 201, 204-205, 211-
        213
    substitutes for, 245
forearm joint
    motions of, 245

gastrocnemius muscle
    actions of, 131, 145, 154, 156,
    160
    substitutes for, 248
gearshift
    moving right upper extremity
    to, 202-205, 212-213
gemelii muscles
    substitutes for, 247
gluteus maximus muscle
    actions of, 145, 184, 231, 233
        in cycling, 154, 158
        in donning shoe, 173, 176
        in driving, 208-209, 215-217,
        219
    substitutes for, 247
gluteus medius muscle
    actions of, 131, 154, 156, 207,
    215
    substitutes for, 247
gluteus minimus muscle
    actions of, 131
    substitutes for, 247
goniometric measurements, 10
    example of, 13
    on videography, 4, 7
gracilis muscle
    actions of, 160
    substitutes for, 247
grasping
    broom, 78
    brush, 39-41
    razor, 25-26

sock, 92-95
grips
    chuck
        three-jaw, 26, 68, 93, 105
        two-jaw, 68, 93, 107
    power, 41, 107

hair
    brushing, 39-55
hamstring muscles
    actions of, 129, 141, 160, 173,
    208-209, 216-219
hand rims
    reaching for, 231-232
hip joint
    anatomy of, 171, 173
    motions of, 247

iliocostalis cervicis muscle, 231
iliopsoas muscle
    actions of, 129, 131, 141, 145,
    184
        in cycling, 154, 160, 165
        in driving, 207-209, 214-215,
        218
    substitutes for, 247
infraspinatus muscle
    actions of, 46, 65-66, 69, 111, 233
    substitutes for, 244
interosseous muscles
    actions of, 26, 41, 78, 112, 120,
    232-234
        in donning shirt, 59, 63, 69-
        70
        in driving, 201, 205, 211, 213
    substitutes for, 246
intervertebral joints, 171
K
knee
    motions of, 248

substitutes for, 245
supraspinatus muscle
    actions of, 65, 69, 81, 111, 201,
    232-233
        in driving, 202, 204, 210-212
    substitutes for, 244
sweeping, 77-90

tensor fasciae latae muscles
    actions of, 129, 160, 207-208, 215
    substitutes for, 247
teres major muscle
    actions of, 28, 46, 119-120, 232
        in donning shirt, 62, 65-66,
        69
        in sweeping, 79, 84
        in tying shoelaces, 111, 114
    substitutes for, 244
teres minor muscle
    actions of, 46, 65, 69, 111, 233
    substitutes for, 244
thoracic vertebrae, 171-172
three-jaw chuck grip, 26, 68, 93,
105
thumb
    motions of, 245-246
tibialis anterior muscle
    actions of, 129, 141, 145, 154,
    160
    substitutes for, 248
tibialis posterior muscle
    actions of, 131, 141, 145, 208
    substitutes for, 248
toes
    motions of, 248
triceps brachii muscle
    actions of, 41, 44, 66, 81, 95, 111,
    232-233
        in driving, 202, 204, 211-212
    substitutes for, 245
trunk
    bringing forward, 173-176

motions of, 249
two-jaw chuck grip, 68, 93, 107
tying shoelaces, 105-116

upper extremity
    analyses of, 21-126
        with lower, 197-226
    left
        dressing, 63-66
        graphing broom handle
        with, 80-81
        reaching with, 81
        in stabilizing bowl, 120-121
        in sweeping, 83-84
    muscles of, 244-246
    right
        drawing broom in with, 79-
        80
        dressing, 60-63
        moving to gearshift, 202-205,
        212-213
        in stirring, 117-120
        in sweeping, 84
upper trapezius muscle
    actions of, 43-44, 118-120, 175,
    230, 232-233
        in donning shirt, 58, 65-66
        in driving, 201-202, 204-205,
        210-213
    substitutes for, 244

vertebrae, 171-172
videography, 4, 7
    with body markers, 9
    use with performance, 11

wheelchair
    propelling, 229-241
wrist
    motions of, 245

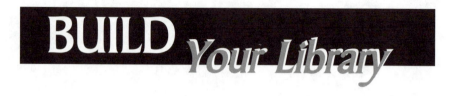

BUILD *Your Library*

This book and many others on numerous different topics are available from SLACK Incorporated. For further information or a copy of our latest catalog, contact us at:

**Professional Book Division
SLACK Incorporated
6900 Grove Road
Thorofare, NJ 08086 USA
Telephone: 1-856-848-1000
1-800-257-8290
Fax: 1-856-853-5991
E-mail: orders@slackinc.com
www.slackbooks.com**

We accept most major credit cards and checks or money orders in US dollars drawn on a US bank. Most orders are shipped within 72 hours.

Contact us for information on recent releases, forthcoming titles, and bestsellers. If you have a comment about this title or see a need for a new book, direct your correspondence to the Editorial Director at the above address.

Thank you for your interest and we hope you found this work beneficial.